MW01000839

NURSING REVIEW AND RESOURCE MANUAL

Psychiatric–Mental Health Nursing

Published by American Nurses Credentialing Center
Authors: Elizabeth Arnold, PhD, RN, PMHCNS-BC
Karan Kverno, PhD, PMHNP-BC, PMHCNS-BC

CONTINUING EDUCATION SOURCE
NURSING CERTIFICATION REVIEW MANUAL
CLINICAL PRACTICE RESOURCE

3RD EDITION

Library of Congress Cataloging-in-Publication Data

Arnold, Elizabeth.
  Psychiatric-mental health nursing : review and resource manual / by Elizabeth Arnold & Karan
Kverno. – 3rd ed.
       p. ; cm.
  Includes bibliographical references and index.
  ISBN-13: 978-1-935213-01-7
  ISBN-10: 1-935213-01-6
  1. Psychiatric nursing–Outlines, syllabi, etc. 2. Psychiatric nursing–Examinations–Study guides. I.
Kverno, Karan. II. American Nurses Credentialing Center. III. Title.
  [DNLM: 1. Psychiatric Nursing–Outlines. WY 18.2 A753p 2009]
  RC440.A757 2009
  616.89'0231–dc22   2009025851

The American Nurses Credentialing Center (ANCC), a subsidiary of the American Nurses Association
(ANA), provides individuals and organizations throughout the nursing profession with the resources they
need to achieve practice excellence. ANCC's internationally renowned credentialing programs certify
nurses in specialty practice areas; recognize healthcare organizations for promoting safe, positive work
environments through the Magnet Recognition Program® and the Pathway to Excellence ® Program;
and accredit providers of continuing nursing education. In addition, ANCC's Institute for Credentialing
Innovation provides leading-edge information and education services and products to support its core
credentialing programs.

ISBN 13: 978-1-935213-01-7   ISBN 10: 1-935213-01-6
© 2009 American Nurses Credentialing Center.
8515 Georgia Ave., Suite 400
Silver Spring, MD 20910
All rights reserved.

Psychiatric–Mental Health Review and Resource Manual, 3rd Edition

SEPTEMBER 2009

Please direct your comments and/or queries to: revmanuals@ana.org

The healthcare services delivery system is a volatile marketplace demanding superior knowledge, clinical skills, and competencies from all registered nurses. Nursing autonomy of practice and nurse career marketability and mobility in the new century hinge on affirming the profession's formative philosophy, which places a priority on a lifelong commitment to the principles of education and professional development. The knowledge base of nursing theory and practice is expanding, and while care has been taken to ensure the accuracy and timeliness of the information presented in the **Psychiatric–Mental Health Nursing Review and Resource Manual, 3rd Edition,** clinicians are advised to always verify the most current national guidelines and recommendations and to practice in accordance with professional standards of care used with regard to the unique circumstances that apply in each practice situation. In addition, the editors wish to note that provision of information in this text does not imply an endorsement of any particular products, procedures or services.

Therefore, the authors, editors, American Nurses Association (ANA), American Nurses Association's Publishing (ANP), American Nurses Credentialing Center (ANCC), and the Institute for Credentialing Innovation cannot accept responsibility for errors or omissions, or for any consequences or liability, injury, and/or damages to persons or property from application of the information in this manual and make no warranty, express or implied, with respect to the contents of the **Psychiatric–Mental Health Nursing Review and Resource Manual, 3rd Edition.**

Published by:
American Nurses Credentialing Center
The Institute for Credentialing Innovation
8515 Georgia Avenue, Suite 400
Silver Spring, MD 20910-3402
www.nursecredentialing.org

Introduction to the Continuing Education (CE) Contact Hour Application Process for *Psychiatric–Mental Health Nursing Review and Resource Manual,* *3rd Edition*

The Institute for Credentialing Innovation now offers the continuing education contact hours for this manual online at www.NursingWorld.org, the American Nurses Association's Web site. This process involves answering approximately 25–30 questions that test knowledge of the information contained within this manual. The continuing education contact hours can be completed at any time and a certificate can be printed from the Web site immediately upon successful completion of the test.

After studying the manual and given an online multiple-choice test, the exam candidate will be able to:

1. Pass the posttest with at least 75% of the answers correct.
2. Select responses to test questions based on key principles, standards of practice, and theoretical basis of nursing practice.
3. Choose accepted therapeutic interventions in answering questions related to quality nursing practice.
4. Utilize direct and indirect professional role responsibilities and applications regarding nursing practice in answering test questions.

Upon completion of this manual *and* the online CE test, a nurse can receive a total of 21 continuing education contact hours at a price of $42, only $2 per CE. (ANA members receive a discount on CEs.) **The entire process—online test and evaluation form—must be completed by December 31, 2011 in order to receive credit.** To begin the process, please e-mail **revmanuals@ana.org.** Your patience with this process is greatly appreciated.

Inquiries or Comments

If you have any questions about the CE contact hours, please e-mail The Institute at revmanuals@ana.org. You may also mail any comments to Editor/Project Manager, at the address listed below.

Duplicate CE Certificates

Once you have successfully passed the CE test on NursingWorld, you may go back and re-print your certificate as often as you wish.

Conflicts of Interest

A conflict of interest occurs when an individual has an opportunity to affect educational content about health-care products or services of a commercial company with which she/he has a financial relationship.

The planners and presenters of this CNE activity have disclosed no relevant financial relationships with any commercial companies pertaining to this activity.

The Institute for Credentialing Innovation
American Nurses Credentialing Center
Attn: Editor/Project Manager
8515 Georgia Avenue, Suite 400
Silver Spring, MD 20910-3492
Fax: (301) 628-5342

The American Nurses Association Center for Continuing Education and Professional Development is accredited as a provider of continuing nursing education by the American Nurses Credentialing Center's Commission on Accreditation.

ANA is approved by the California Board of Registered Nursing, Provider Number 6178.

Contents

Psychiatric–Mental Health Nursing Review and Resource Manual

3RD EDITION

Taking the Certification Examination

When you sign up to take a national certification exam, you will be instructed to go online and review the testing and review handbook (www.nursecredentialing.org/documents/certification/application/generaltestingandreviewhandbook.aspx). Review it carefully and be sure to bookmark the site so you can refer to it frequently. It contains information on test content and sample questions. This is critical information; it will give you insight into the nature of the test. The agency will send you information about the test site; keep this in a safe place until needed.

GENERAL SUGGESTIONS FOR PREPARING FOR THE EXAM

Step One: Control Your Anxiety

Everyone experiences anxiety when faced with taking the certification exam.
- Remember, your program was designed to prepare you to take this exam.
- Your instructors took a similar exam, and have probably talked to students who took exams more recently, so they know how to help you prepare.
- Taking a review course or setting up your own study plan will help you feel more confident about taking the exam.

Step Two: Do Not Listen to Gossip About the Exam

A large volume of information exists about the tests based on reports from people who have taken the exams in the past. Because information from the testing facilities is limited, it is hard to ignore this gossip.

- Remember that gossip about the exam that you hear from others is not verifiable.
- Because this gossip is based on the imperfect memory of people in a very stressful situation, it may not be very accurate.
- People tend to remember those items testing content with which they are less comfortable; for instance, those with a limited background in women's health may say that the exam was "all women's health." In fact, the exam blueprint ensures that the exam covers multiple content areas without overemphasizing any one.

Step Three: Set Reasonable Expectations for Yourself

- Do not expect to know everything.
- Do not try to know everything in great detail.
- You do not need a perfect score to pass the exam.
- The exam is designed for a beginner level—it is testing readiness for entry-level practice.
- Learn the general rules, not the exceptions.
- The most likely diagnoses will be on the exam, not questions on rare diseases or atypical cases.
- Think about the most likely presentation and most common therapy.

Step Four: Prepare Mentally and Physically

- While you are getting ready to take the exam, take good physical care of yourself.
- Get plenty of sleep, exercise, and eat well while preparing for the exam.
- These things are especially important while you are studying and immediately before you take the exam.

Step Five: Access Current Knowledge

General Content
You will be given a list of general topics that will be on the exam when you register to take the exam. In addition, examine the table of contents of this book and the test content outline, available at www.nursecredentialing.org/cert/TCOs.html.
- What content do you need to know?
- How well do you know these subjects?

Take a Review Course
- Taking a review course is an excellent method of assessing your knowledge of the content that will be included in the exam.
- If you plan to take a review course, take it well before the exam so you will have plenty of time to master any areas of weakness the course uncovers.

- If you are prepared for the exam, you will not hear anything new in the course. You will be familiar with everything that is taught.
- If some topics in the review course are new to you, concentrate on these in your studies.
- People have a tendency to study what they know; it is rewarding to study something and feel a mastery of it! Unfortunately, this will not help you master unfamiliar content. Be sure to use a review course to identify your areas of strength and weakness, then concentrate on the weaknesses.

Depth of Knowledge
How much do you need to know about a subject?
- You cannot know everything about a topic.
- Remember that the depth of knowledge required to pass the exam is for entry-level performance.
- Study the information sent to you from the testing agency, what you were taught in school, what is covered in this text, and the general guidelines given in this chapter.
- Look at practice tests designed for the exam. Practice tests for other exams will not be helpful.
- Consult your class notes or clinical diagnosis and management textbook for the major points about a disease. Additional reference books can be found online at www.nursecredentialing.org/cert/refs.html.
- For example, with regard to medications, know the drug categories and the major medications in each. Assume all drugs in a category are generally alike, and then focus on the differences among common drugs. Know the most important indications, contraindications, and side effects. Emphasize safety. The questions usually do not require you to know the exact dosage of a drug.

Step Six: Institute a Systematic Study Plan

Develop Your Study Plan
- Write up a formal plan of study.
  - Include topics for study, timetable, resources, and methods of study that work for you.
  - Decide whether you want to organize a study group or work alone.
  - Schedule regular times to study.
  - Avoid cramming; it is counterproductive. Try to schedule your study periods in 1-hour increments.
- Identify resources to use for studying. To prepare for the examination, you should have the following materials on your shelf:
  - A good pathophysiology text.
  - This review book.
  - A physical assessment text.
  - Your class notes.
  - Other important sources, including: information from the testing facility, a clinical diagnosis textbook, favorite journal articles, notes from a review course, and practice tests.
  - Know the important national standards of care for major illnesses.
  - Consult the bibliography on the test blueprint. When studying less familiar material, it is helpful to study using the same references that the testing center uses.

- Study the body systems from head to toe.
- The exams emphasize health promotion, assessment, differential diagnosis, and plan of care for common problems.
- You will need to know facts and be able to interpret and analyze this information utilizing critical thinking.

Personalize Your Study Plan
- How do you learn best?
  - If you learn best by listening or talking, attend a review course or discuss topics with a colleague.
- Read everything the test facility sends you as soon as you receive it and several times during your preparation period. It will give you valuable information to help guide your study.
- Have a specific place with good lighting set aside for studying. Find a quiet place with no distractions. Assemble your study materials.

Implement Your Study Plan
You must have basic content knowledge. In addition, you must be able to use this information to think critically and make decisions based on facts.
- Refer to your study plan regularly.
- Stick to your schedule.
- Take breaks when you get tired.
- If you start procrastinating, get help from a friend or reorganize your study plan.
- It is not necessary to follow your plan rigidly. Adjust as you learn where you need to spend more time.
- Memorize the basics of the content areas you will be required to know.

Focus on General Material
- Most of what you need to know is basic material that does not require constant updating.
- You do not need to worry about the latest information being published as you are studying for the exam. Remember, it can take 6 to 12 months for new information to be incorporated into test questions.

Pace Your Studying
- Stop studying for the examination when you are starting to feel overwhelmed and look at what is bothering you, then make changes.
- Break overwhelming tasks into smaller tasks that you know you can do.
- Stop and take breaks while studying.

Work With Others
- Talk with classmates about your preparation for the exam.
- Keep in touch with classmates, and help each other stick to your study plans.
- If your classmates start having anxiety attacks, do not let their anxiety affect you. Walk away if you need to.
- Do not believe bad stories you hear about other people's experiences with previous exams.
- Remember, you know as much as anyone about what will be on the next exam!

Consider a Study Group
- Study groups can provide practice in analyzing cases, interpreting questions, and critical thinking.
  - You can discuss a topic and take turns presenting cases for the group to analyze.
  - Study groups can also provide moral support and help you continue studying.

Step Seven: Strategies Immediately Before the Exam

Final Preparation Suggestions
- Use practice exams when studying to get accustomed to the exam format and time restrictions.
  - Many books that are labeled as review books are simply a collection of examination questions.
  - If you have test anxiety, such practice tests may help alleviate the anxiety.
  - Practice tests can help you learn to judge the time it should take you to complete the exam.
  - Practice tests are useful for gaining experience in analyzing questions.
  - Books of questions may not uncover the gaps in your knowledge that a more systematic content review text will reveal.
  - If you feel that you don't know enough about a topic, refer to a text to learn more. After you feel that you have learned the topic, practice questions are a wonderful tool to help improve your test-taking skill.
- Know your test-taking style.
  - Do you rush through the exam without reading the questions thoroughly?
  - Do you get stuck and dwell on a question for a long time?
  - You should spend about 45 to 60 seconds per question and finish with time to review the questions you were not sure about.
  - Be sure to read the question completely, including all four answer choices. Choice "a" may be good, but "d" may be best.

The Night Before the Exam
- Be prepared to get to the exam on time.
  - Know the test site location and how long it takes to get there.
  - Take a "dry run" beforehand to make sure you know how to get to the testing site, if necessary.
  - Get good night's sleep.
  - Eat sensibly.
  - Avoid alcohol the night before.
  - Assemble the required material—two forms of identification, admission card, pencil, and watch. Both IDs must match the name on the application, and one photo ID is preferred. Bring tissues, antacid chews, hard candy, and anything you might want in your pocket.
- Know the exam room rules.
  - You will be given scratch paper, which will be collected at the end of the exam.
  - Nothing else is allowed in the exam room.
  - You will be required to put papers, backpacks, etc., in a corner of the room, or in a locker.

- No water or food will be allowed.
  - You will be allowed to walk to a water fountain and go to the bathroom one at a time.

The Day of the Exam

- Get there early. If you are late, you may not be admitted.
- Think positively. You have studied hard and are well-prepared.
- Remember your anxiety reduction strategies.

Specific Tips for Dealing With Anxiety

Test anxiety is a specific type of anxiety. Symptoms include upset stomach, sweaty palms, tachycardia, trouble concentrating, and a feeling of dread. But there are ways to cope with test anxiety.

- There is no substitute for being well-prepared.
- Practice relaxation techniques.
- Avoid alcohol, excess coffee, caffeine, and any new medications that might sedate you, dull your senses, or make you feel agitated.
- Take a few deep breaths and concentrate on the task at hand.

Focus on Specific Test-Taking Skills

To do well on the exam, you need good test-taking skills in addition to knowledge of the content and ability to use critical thinking.

All Certification Exams Are Multiple Choice

- Multiple choice tests have specific rules for test construction.
- A multiple choice question consists of three parts: the information (or stem), the question, and the four possible answers (one correct and three distracters).
- Careful analysis of each part is necessary. Read the entire question before answering.
- Practice your test-taking skills by analyzing the practice questions in this book and on the ANCC website.

Analyze the Information Given

- Do not assume you have more information than is given.
- Do not overanalyze.
- Remember, the writer of the question assumes this is all of the information needed to answer the question.
- If information is not given, it is not relevant and will not affect the answer.
- Do not make the question more complicated than it is.

What Kind of Question Is Asked?

- Are you supposed to recall a fact, apply facts to a situation, or understand and differentiate between options?
  - Read the question thinking about what the writer is asking.
  - Look for key words or phrases that lead you (see Figure 1–1). These help determine what kind of answer the question requires.

Figure 1-1. Examples of Key Words and Phrases

- avoid
- best
- except
- not
- initial
- first
- contributing to
- appropriate
- most
- significant
- likely
- of the following
- most consistent with

Read All of the Answers
- If you are absolutely certain that answer "a" is correct as you read it, mark it, but read the rest of the question so you do not trick yourself into missing a better answer.
- If you are absolutely sure answer "a" is wrong, cross it off or make a note on your scratch paper and continue reading the question.
- After reading the entire question, go back, analyze the question, and select the best answer.
- Do not jump ahead.
- If the question asks you for an assessment, the best answer will be an assessment. Do not be distracted by an intervention that sounds appropriate.
- If the question asks you for an intervention, do not answer with an assessment.
- When two answer choices sound very good, the best one is usually the least expensive, least invasive way to achieve the goal. For example, if your answer choices include a physical exam maneuver or imaging, the physical exam maneuver is probably the better choice provided it will give the information needed.
- If the answers include two options that are the opposite of each other, one of the two is probably the correct answer.
- When numeric answers cover a wide range, a number in the middle is more likely to be correct.
- Watch out for distracters that are correct but do not answer the question, combine true and false information, or contain a word or phrase that is similar to the correct answer.
- Err on the side of caution.

Only One Answer Can Be Correct
- When more than one suggested answer is correct, you must identify the one that best answers the question asked.
- If you cannot choose between two answers, you have a 50% chance of getting it right if you guess.

Avoid Changing Answers
- Change an answer only if you have a compelling reason, such as you remembered something additional, or you understand the question better after rereading it.
- People change to a wrong answer more often than to a right answer.

Time Yourself to Complete the Whole Exam

- Do not spend a large amount of time on one question.
- If you cannot answer a question quickly, mark it and continue the exam.
- If time is left at the end, return to the difficult questions.
- Make educated guesses by eliminating the obviously wrong answers and choosing a likely answer even if you are not certain.
- Trust your instinct.
- Answer every question. There is no penalty for a wrong answer.
- Occasionally a question will remind you of something that helps you with a question earlier in the test. Look back at that question to see if what you are remembering affects how you would answer that question.

About the Certification Exams

The American Nurses Credentialing Center Computerized Exam

The ANCC examination is given only as a computer exam, and each exam is different. The order of the questions is scrambled for every test, so even if two people are taking the same exam, the questions will be in a different order. The exam consists of 175 multiple-choice questions.

- 150 of the 175 questions are part of the test and how you answer will count toward your score; 25 are included to refine questions and will not be scored. You will not know which ones count, so treat all questions the same.
- You will need to know how to use a mouse, scroll by either clicking arrows on the scroll bar or using the up and down arrow keys, and perform other basic computer tasks.
- The exam does not require computer expertise.
- However, if you are not comfortable with using a computer, you should practice using a mouse and computer beforehand so you do not waste time on the mechanics of using the computer.

Know what to expect during the test.
- Each ANCC test question is independent of the other questions.
  - For each case study, there is only one question. This means that a correct answer on any question does not depend on the correct answer to any other question.
  - Each question has four possible answers. There are no questions asking for combinations of correct answers (such as "a and c") or multiple-multiples.
- You can skip a question and go back to it at the end of the exam.
- You cannot mark key words in the question or right or wrong answers. If you want to do this, use the scratch paper.
- You will get your results immediately, and a grade report will be provided upon leaving the testing site.

Other Resources

- ANCC website: www.nursecredentialing.org
- ANA website: www.nursesbooks.org. Catalog of ANA nursing scope and standards publications and other titles that may be listed on your test content outline
- National Guideline Clearinghouse: www.ngc.gov

Theories and Frameworks for Psychiatric Nursing Practice

Elizabeth Arnold, PhD, RN, PMHCNS-BC

Chapter 2 reviews common theoretical frameworks used in psychiatric–mental health nursing. Included in the chapter are descriptions of theories of personality development, theory frameworks from psychology, and nursing theory that guide the therapeutic treatment of individuals suffering from mental disorders. An explanation of differentiated practice roles and certification is included.

THEORIES OF PERSONALITY DEVELOPMENT

Freud's Theory of Psychosexual Development

Freud conceptually explained personality development in terms of psychosexual stages. He maintained that a child's personality naturally evolves through a variety of age-related, sequential stages of development, each focused on a primary erogenous zone (body part). If the child successfully negotiates the associated life issues at the appropriate stage, personality develops normally. If these life issues are not successfully resolved during the appropriate developmental stage, because of parental overindulgence or frustration, a person becomes "fixated" at that psychosexual developmental stage. This fixation will significantly affect his or her adult personality in negative ways. Freud's stages of psychosexual development (see Table 2–1) include

- *Oral stage (birth to 18 months).* The erogenous zone in the oral stage is the mouth, which infants and toddlers use to explore their world, and then to communicate through words. Fixation behaviors include alcoholism, overeating, overdependence on others.
- *Anal stage (18 months to 3 years),* during which the anus is the child's most sensitive erogenous zone as the toddler learns to control elimination of body wastes through toilet training. The unsuccessful resolution of the anal stage can result in a personality "fixation" on obsessive behaviors and problems with authority figures.
- *Phallic stage (3 to 5 years of age),* which represents the most critical psychosexual conflict in Freud's developmental model. Here the erogenous zone is the genital region as the child begins to explore sexual differences between girls and boys. The conflict is labeled the Oedipus complex in boys, and the Electra complex in girls. These complexes lead, according to Freudian theory, to normal differentiation of male and female personalities. Fixation at this psychosexual stage of development can result in uncertainty about one's identity as a male or female and affect a person's capacity to engage in a close, loving relationship.
- *Latency period (6 to 12 years of age).* Freud did not consider latency to be a psychosexual stage of development but rather a period of dormancy in which the child's libidinal energy is repressed and diverted into asexual activities such as athletics, school activities, and same-sex friendships.
- *Genital stage (12 to 15 years of age)* focuses on the genitals as the primary erogenous zone. As the teenager develops mature sexual characteristics, his or her sexual interests focus on the opposite sex. Successful negotiation of life issues associated with the genital phase form the central foundation for mature sexual relationships.

Freud did not describe stage development in adulthood.

Table 2-1. Freud's Stages of Psychosexual Development

Stage	Age Range	Zone	Developmental Task
Oral	Birth to 18 months	Mouth	Establishing trusting dependence
Anal	18 months to 3 years	Anus	Development of self-control; feelings of autonomy
Phallic	3 to 5 years	Genital area	Establishing sexual role identity
Latency	6 to 12 years	Period when sexual drive is dormant	Group identification
Genital	12 to 15 years	Genital area	Development of social control over instincts

Erikson's Theory of Psychosocial Development

Erik Erikson described personality development using psychosocial stages. Unlike Freud, Erikson maintained that personality development does not end with adolescence, but continues to develop from birth through death. He broadened Freud's conceptualization of personality development to include social and cultural influences on psychosocial personality development. According to Erikson, the epigenetic stages of personality development are present at birth, but will unfold according to a planned, sequential, age-related schema that incorporates cultural and social values.

Each stage is characterized by a particular psychosocial crisis involving a specific developmental task that builds on previous stages, and points the way for subsequent stages. This task must be achieved for a healthy transition to the next phase of development. While ideally the ego should sequentially resolve the appropriate psychosocial crisis for each developmental stage, Erikson proposes that outcomes of stage development are not fixed. They can be modified by later positive experiences and/or challenges to the ego. Erikson also identified a specific virtue or strength associated with each developmental stage.

Erikson's Eight Stages of Man

Stage One: Trust vs. Mistrust (Birth to 1 year)
- Virtue or strength: Hope
- Corresponds to Freud's sensory/oral stage of development
- Quality of the primary caregiver relationship has a profound effect on the child's ability to balance trust with mistrust
- Needs must be met for basic core of trust to develop

Stage Two: Autonomy vs. Shame and Doubt (1–3 years of age)
- Virtue or strength: Willpower
- Corresponds to Freud's anal/muscular stage of development
- Child learns sense of self; self-consciousness is associated with doubt
- Mastering skills involving the learning of control over bodily functions; holding on and letting go; what is the child's and what is someone else's; where he or she begins and ends is primary
- Learning limits and what is permissible in the environment helps develop important skills related to the will
- Task is for child to learn these things and parent to teach these things successfully and without excessive shame or doubt
- Autonomy = sense of rightful dignity and lawful independence
- Shame = self-consciousness; one is visible and not ready to be visible; being "shamed" leads to repressed rage and defiance
- Doubt = brother of shame; fear of being attacked or overpowered

Stage Three: Initiative vs. Guilt (3–6 years of age)
- Strength or virtue: Purpose
- Corresponds to Freud's genital/phallic/Oedipal stage of development
- Guilt = sense of badness

- Task of identification with same-sex parent to make oneself endearing to opposite-sex parent
- Child takes initiative in creating play roles observed in the adults around him or her
- Child begins to take on social role identification consistent with his or her gender. Natural sexual curiosity needs to be satisfied; questions about where babies come from and masturbation are normal.
- Parents have to teach children what is appropriate without inflicting sense of badness about themselves, sex, or their bodies

Stage Four: Industry vs. Inferiority (6–12 years of age)
- Strength or virtue: Competence
- Corresponds to Freud's latency stage of development
- Development of multiple skills, which create the sense of industry and accomplishment
- Experience success and failure; feelings of inadequacy and inferiority occur when competence is not achievable
- Manual and social dexterity
- Need good role models outside the family (e.g., teachers, scout leaders)
- To avoid a sense of inferiority, child must be exposed to multiple arenas to discover his or her best skills
- "Hero worship" and same-sex crushes common

Stage Five: Identity vs. Role Confusion (12–18 years of age; puberty and adolescence)
- Strength or virtue: Fidelity
- Most important stage according to Erikson
- "Who am I … how am I different and separate from my family of origin…what is my role in society?"
- Emancipation from parents and development of independence
- Definition of sexual identity and role; straight, gay, popular, sexy
- Gangs and cliques prevail; need for sense of belonging
- Conflict of biological readiness for sexual expression vs. cultural conventions and need for more emotional maturity
- Developing a personal philosophy of life, morals, and values

Stage Six: Intimacy vs. Isolation (young adulthood)
- Strength or virtue: Love
- Builds on a sense of identity by expanding it to include relationships with others
- Mate selection
- Development of mutually satisfying relationships through marriage and friends
- Starting a family and keeping relationship commitments
- Experiencing a sense of intimacy with partners, friends, companions

Stage Seven: Generativity vs. Stagnation (middle adulthood)
- Strength or virtue: Care
- Creating meaningful work
- Establishing and guiding the next generation
- Contributing to the betterment of society
- Coping with life changes—midlife crisis, which creates the need for new meanings and purpose

- Stagnation = self-absorption
- Socializing vs. sexualizing in human relationships

Stage Eight: Ego Integrity vs. Despair (maturity/old age)
- Strength or virtue: Wisdom
- Life review as the individual looks back on his or her life
- Feeling life has meaning and one has made a meaningful, vital contribution = integrity
- Feeling that life has had little meaning and reflecting on perceived failures = despair
- Can accept death as a part and completion of life

Jean Piaget's Theory of Cognitive Development

Jean Piaget's theory of cognitive development is perhaps the best-known theory in cognitive developmental psychology. He was a Swiss child psychologist who believed that learning was an active, dynamic process comprising four successive developmental stages of adaptation leading to increasingly complex levels of organization (principle of equilibration). Piaget proposed that a child's physiological and psychological maturation together with their social environment played a significant role in a child's cognitive development. Thus, interaction with the social environment plays an important role in the development of intellectual competence. Piaget proposed that children develop cognitive structures, which he labeled schemas, to help them learn about and understand their environment. These schemas create increasingly complex understanding through complementary processes that Piaget named assimilation, accommodation, and organization.

- *Assimilation* is the process of using and transforming environmental data so that they can be placed in preexisting cognitive structures. Example: Infant is able to transfer the same sucking schema used to suck from the breast to suck successfully from a bottle.
- *Accommodation* is the process of developing a new mental schema, which the infant uses when the new information does not fit into established cognitive structures. In this case, the schema itself changes to accommodate the new information. Example: Infant needs to modify the sucking schema developed by sucking on the breast or bottle to learning to drink from a glass.
- *Organization* is the natural process by which the child learns to organize information into related, interconnected structures.

Piaget describes four stages of cognitive development:
- *Sensorimotor* (infancy). In this stage, the child learns about the environment through motor activity. Knowledge of the world (environment) takes place through direct physical interactions and experiences with touching and feeling objects. Physical mobility allows the child to explore and gain new intellectual knowledge.
- *Pre-operational stage* (toddler and early childhood). In this stage of cognitive development, the child begins to incorporate the use of symbols as language use emerges and the child is able to express thoughts verbally. The child acquires representational skills and mental imagery emerges. However, thinking occurs in a nonreversible manner; thought processes are predominantly egocentric and concrete so the child is only able to think about things from his or her perspective.

- *Concrete operational stage* (elementary school age >7 years through early adolescence). In this stage, the child demonstrates more complex thinking skills through manipulation of symbols associated with concrete objects, and is able to classify objects using a variety of criteria. The child is able to take into account more than one perspective, but is not able to consider all of the logically possible outcomes. As concrete operational thinking develops, the child is able to conduct mental activities that are reversible, such as combining, subtracting, dividing, sorting, or seeing the connection between a nickel and two dimes representing the same 25 cents as a quarter.
- *Formal operational stage* (adolescence and adulthood). In this stage, there is a significant cognitive shift that allows for the logical use of symbols related to abstract concepts. Children in the formal operations stage can formulate hypotheses and reason theoretically, without referring to concrete objects. They can think through and problem-solve issues at an abstract level. They have the capacity to appreciate a wide range of viewpoints. Not all adolescents or adults reach the formal operation stage.

Developmental delays observed in a child's cognitive development sometimes are associated with meeting physical maturation milestones and educational expectancies. In addition to psychosocial benchmarks, areas of concern can include "attention and activity regulation; speech and language; play; motor skills; bladder and bowel control; and scholastic attainments, particularly in reading, spelling, and mathematics" (Goodman & Scott, 2005, p. 5).

Lawrence Kohlberg's Moral Development Theory

Lawrence Kohlberg (Kohlberg, Levine, & Hewer, 1983) developed a sequential model of moral development comprised of three levels, pre-conventional, conventional, and post-conventional, and six stages of moral reasoning.

Pre-Conventional
- *Stage one: Obedience and punishment driven.* Moral reasoning and decision-making is based solely on the consequence that taking one action over another entails. There is no recognition of the needs or rights of others. Commonly found in children.
- *Stage two: Self-interest driven.* Moral reasoning and behavior is based on the individual's perception of what is best for him- or herself in the situation. Beginning token awareness of the needs of others, but only in relation to how it would benefit oneself.

Conventional Levels (Found in adolescents and adults)
- *Stage three: Interpersonal accord and conformity driven.* Moral reasoning and decision-making reflects the person's perception of the social approval or disapproval of a moral action. The person evaluates the rightness or wrongness of a behavior according to the dictates of personalized social approval and acts accordingly.
- *Stage four: Authority and social order obedience driven.* Moral reasoning and decision-making begins to transcend individual interpretations of the meaning of behavior. There is awareness and acceptance of more universal ideas of what is right and wrong. Kohlberg suggests that most people's moral reasoning rests at stage four.

Post-Conventional Level

The post-conventional level of moral reasoning is referred to as the principled level. It incorporates differences in individual values with social understandings, resulting in a broader and deeper examination of the rightness or wrongness of value-laden behaviors.

- *Stage five: Social contract driven.* Moral reasoning and decision-making reflect a self-determining understanding of different values and opinions measured against social laws. The person is able to draw moral conclusions about behaviors based on what is best for the general well-being of all concerned in a particular situation.
- *Stage six: Universal ethical principles driven.* Moral reasoning and decision-making is based on abstract reasoning of what is justice in a particular situation. The person acts because something is morally right in and of itself, and not in relation to the expectations of others, or of accepted social values. Most people do not achieve stage six of moral reasoning.

THEORIES FROM PSYCHOLOGY

Psychoanalytic Theory

Although psychoanalytic approaches are no longer regularly used in today's managed care environment, many of the concepts remain relevant knowledge for psychiatric nurses. Psychoanalytic theory was initially developed by Sigmund Freud and is based on the premise that most behavior is unconsciously motivated. Psychoanalytic theory proposes that helping patients trace these unconscious contributors to current behavior patterns and relationships enables people to better understand their dysfunctional patterns of relating, and correct their behavior. Freud also developed psychosexual stages of personality development and described the structure of personality.

Freud

Freud defined the personality as consisting of three major systems: the id, the ego, and the superego. Freud believed that the id, the ego, and the superego are in frequent conflict. Discordant interaction among the three systems can lead to maladjusted behavior. Internal conflicts create anxiety, which occurs when the ego cannot successfully mediate between the id and the superego. The ego uses mostly unconscious defense mechanisms to protect the person from experiencing anxiety.

- The *id* refers to man's primitive drives or instinctual energy—those associated with raw pleasure, hunger, sex, and aggression. The id operates according to the "pleasure principle," expecting immediate gratification of these drives without thought to the reality of a situation.
- The *ego* is the part of the personality in contact with reality. The ego's primary function is to mediate between the instinctual impulses and the environment. The ego functions as a mediator to protect the person from acting solely on instinctual primitive drives, while at the same time providing a reality check for superego rigidity. Sometimes referred to as the personality's "executive function," the ego is associated with a person's higher cognitive functions of thoughtful reflection and learning.

- The *superego* emerges later, representing morality and the ethical standards of society. The superego evolves when the individual has the capacity to identify with and internalize the prohibitions and demands of parent figures, primarily in response to rewards and punishments. The superego consists of two elements: conscience, which prevents individuals from doing morally wrong actions, and ego ideal, which motivates individuals to perform at higher moral levels. The superego can be in conflict with the id and ego as it fulfills its functions of inhibiting the expression of id impulses, persuading the ego to substitute moralist goals for realistic ones, or strives for perfection.

Freud believed that behavior is heavily influenced by unconscious motivation and anxiety. He was the first theorist to introduce the concept of the unconscious, which he contended was key to understanding hidden mental processes that govern behavior. Therapeutic interventions are designed to help the client bring into conscious awareness those unconscious conflicts that the client is still acting on in the present. Freud was the first theorist to describe transference, countertransference, and resistance. These psychological processes, along with defense mechanisms (see Chapter 3), can sabotage a relationship. This often occurs without the individual having any real recognition of why he or she is feeling and reacting to the other in a manner that has little to do with the reality of the current situation.

- *Transference* relates to a patient's unconsciously activated experience of negative and positive emotions, conflicts, and attitudes from the past in a current therapeutic relationship.
- *Countertransference* relates to unconsciously activated reactions of the helping person or therapist towards a client or patient, stemming from unresolved conflicts in past relationships.
- *Resistance* is anything that disrupts the progression of the therapeutic alliance or working on therapeutic issues.

Interpersonal Psychodynamic Theory

Harry Stack Sullivan's theoretical model focused on anxiety as being a consequence of faulty social interactions. Individuals begin to develop personifications of self and others as the "bad me," the "good me," and the "not me" based on interpersonal interactions with important people in their lives. The "good me" represents those aspects of self that people like about themselves and are willing to share with others. The *"good me"* produces very little anxiety. The "bad me" represents the parts of self that a person does not like and is reluctant to share with others. The *"bad me"* creates anxiety. The *"not me"* represents those aspects of self that are so anxiety-provoking that the person does not consider them to be a part of him- or herself. This part of self exists primarily in the unconscious. Individuals cope with the anxiety produced by undesired traits through *selective inattention*. Sullivan's description of *parataxic distortion* refers to a person's fantasy perception of a person's attributes, for example, describing a new love relationship as "a perfect match" without considering important personality differences. The concept is similar to Freud's explanation of transference and counter-transference.

Sullivan considered the interpersonal relationship as the keystone of therapeutic intervention. Hildegard Peplau patterned her theoretical approach to nursing interventions with psychiatric patients on Sullivan's theory, as did Gerald Klerman Interpersonal Psychodynamic Theory (IPT) model for the treatment of depression.

Behaviorism

Behavioral theory, sometimes referred to as behaviorism, is based on the concept that reinforced behaviors are more likely to recur. Rather than considering underlying conflicts hidden in the subconscious, behavioral theorists propose that by changing the environmental cues that reinforce a behavior, one can change the behavior. The patient's internal state or frame of reference is not a focus of treatment. Changing the environmental cues in a systematic manner is referred to as conditioning. There are two types of conditioning: classical conditioning and operant conditioning.

- *Classical conditioning* refers to a process developed by Ivan Pavlov, which first pairs a naturally occurring stimulus with a response, and then pairs a previously neutral stimulus with the naturally occurring stimulus. Over time, the previously neutral stimulus will evoke the same response (conditioned response) without the naturally occurring stimulus. Classical conditioning frameworks have relevance as therapeutic approaches for the treatment of phobias (flooding, desensitization).
- *Operant conditioning* is a method of learning that occurs through rewards and punishments for behavior. B.F. Skinner proposed that changes in behavior occur when a stimulus response is reinforced and the individual is "conditioned" to respond. Operant conditioning associates a behavior with a consequence for that behavior (reinforcer), thereby strengthening, attenuating, or extinguishing the behavioral response as a consequence of the reinforcement. Operant conditioning concepts are the foundation for behavior modification strategies often used in in-patient settings and for children with behavior problems (see Chapter 8).

Cognitive Behavioral Theory

Cognitive behavioral therapy draws from both behavioral and cognitive theory. Cognitive models of emotional response propose that our thoughts strongly influence our feelings and behaviors. It is not how the situation actually is, but how the person perceives it, that is the focus of cognitive behavioral therapy (CBT). Helping patients to change maladaptive thought patterns helps them begin to feel differently about themselves and their situation even though the situation itself remains unchanged. The prototype for cognitive therapy is cognitive behavioral therapy, developed by Aaron Beck. This is an evidence-based therapeutic approach that uses the Socratic method to challenge dysfunctional thinking and broaden a person's perspective to include a number of alternative explanations. The approach uses an inductive format and requires the individual to develop alternative hypotheses that can be questioned, challenged, or supported. The goal of therapy is to help patients become aware of the distorted thinking patterns that interfere with functional living and personal satisfaction.

Humanistic Theory

Human Needs Theory
Abraham Maslow described a hierarchy of needs beginning with the most basic physiologic needs. Individuals must be able to meet their needs at their most basic level before progressing to the next level. As each need level is satisfied, the individual is able to move on to the next level. He referred to the first four levels as deficit need levels, meaning that if these needs are not met, the individual is not able to realize his or her full potential because

attention is focused on meeting lower needs. For example, a person deprived of food or water cannot focus on finding friends or feeling a sense of community because she or he is coping with basic survival needs.

- *Physiologic needs* include air, food, water, sex, rest, sleep, and avoiding pain.
- *Safety and security needs* include finding a stable, safe environment; job security; and having sufficient financial assets to live with at least minimum comfort.
- *Love and belonging needs* include having friends, a supportive family, and a sense of community.
- *Esteem needs* refer to an individual's need to have the respect of others, and the need for self-respect, which includes feelings of confidence and achievement.
- *Self actualization* is a growth motivation need, which can only be addressed when the deficit needs are taken care of satisfactorily. A self-actualized person is not perfect, but rather is reality- and problem-centered. Self-actualized individuals respect themselves and have a healthy respect for others.

Attachment Theory

John Bowlby (1958) describes a theoretical approach related to emotional attachments. He proposed that attachment behaviors are innate instinctive responses occurring between primary caregiver and child. It is possible to observe attachment behaviors in infants, such as smiling, crying, and clinging. Children learn early in life to discriminate between loving, constant caregivers who are sensitive to their needs and others in their environment. Both primary caregiver and child play an active role in seeking proximity and contact with each other. These early experiences create internal working models important in the development of later social relationships. As the child matures, he or she is able to seek other satisfying attachment figures in his or her environment if early attachments have been favorable experiences. The capacity to form reciprocal affectionate bonds with others has an important effect on a person's emotional life. Maternal deprivation, or loss or threat of loss of important attachment figures is a significant factor in the development of psychopathology.

NURSING THEORY FRAMEWORKS

Nursing Domain

In addition to developmental and psychological theories, a variety of nursing theories assist in explaining the science of human behavior and the therapeutic use of self in the art of providing care to individuals. Nursing theories present a distinctive paradigm (world view) with related concepts that distinguish the nursing profession from other disciplines. Application of nursing models provides a basis and direction for clinical nursing practice, education, and research (Fawcett, 2005). The four components of nursing's paradigm, which are addressed in all theories, include:

- *Person:* The recipient of nursing care. Can refer to an individual, population, or community.
- *Environment:* All of the internal and external contextual factors that form the context of the person in the healthcare situation.

- *Health:* A multidimensional concept referring to quality of life; health status; and well-being of individuals, families, and communities.
- *Nurse:* The licensed professional providing the care.

Florence Nightingale was the first nursing theorist, writing her first works on what constituted nursing in 1860. She insisted that by providing a healthy environment with fresh air, cleanliness, and proper diet, nurses can influence a person's ability to get well again. Since Nightingale's time, a number of nurse theorists have proposed models, beginning in the 1950s, to guide nurses in applying nursing knowledge. Professional nurses should be familiar with major nursing theories and models (Fawcett, 2005). In addition to numerous texts on nursing theory, there are websites dedicated to explaining nursing theory (Nursingtheory.net, 2005).

Classification of Nursing Theories

Nursing theories are classified according to their levels of abstraction, ranging from grand theories to practice theories. *Grand theories* represent the most abstract level of theoretical nursing knowledge. They describe broad concepts relevant to nursing practice and are difficult to test. Listed below are some of the better known grand nursing theorists and the central focus of each theorist's model.

- Imogene King: General Systems Framework—*Goal Attainment*
- Dorothea Orem: *Self-Care Framework*
- Dorothy Johnson: *Behavioral Systems Model*
- Madeleine Leininger: *Culture Care Diversity and Universality*
- Martha Rogers: *Science of Unitary Human Beings*
- Betty Neuman: *Neuman Systems Model*
- Margaret Newman: *Theory of Expanding Consciousness*
- Virginia Henderson: *Basic Principles of Nursing Care*
- Rosemarie Parse: *Theory of Human Becoming*
- Sister Callista Roy: *Adaptation Model*
- Myra Levine: *Conservation Model*
- Joyce Travelbee: *Interpersonal Theory of Nursing*
- Jean Watson: *Theory of Human Science and Human Caring*
- Josephine Paterson and Loretta Zderad: *Humanistic Nursing Theory*

Midrange theories cover more discrete aspects of a phenomenon specific to professional nursing, exploring them in depth rather than exploring the full phenomena of nursing (Marrs & Lowery, 2006). Midrange theories are composed of measurable concepts and propositions, which can be tested. Examples of midrange theory include:

- Kathryn Barnard: *Child Interaction Model*
- Nola Pender: *Health Promotion Model*
- Pamela Reed: *Theory of Self-Transcendence*
- Janet Younger: *Mastery of Stress Theory*

Practice theories are the most concrete level of nursing theory, a specific outline for practice. Practice theories can focus on a single operationalized concept found in a specific population or nursing situation. The steps in the development of a practice theory include factor isolating, factor relating, situation relating, and situation producing control. Practice theories are helpful in a healthcare setting focused on developing evidence-based practice. One example is the Chronic Illness Trajectory Model (Corbin & Strauss, 2000).

Hildegard Peplau: Interpersonal Relationship Theory

Hildegard Peplau's (1988) theory of interpersonal relationships, first developed in 1952, is still considered the cornerstone of psychiatric nursing practice. Her theory draws from developmental, interpersonal, and learning theories, particularly the constructs presented by Harry Stack Sullivan.

Peplau viewed nursing as "an educative instrument, a maturing force that aims to promote forward movement of personality in the direction of creative, constructive, productive, personal, and community living" (p. 16). She described the phases of the therapeutic nurse–patient relationship, and identified six common roles that nurses assume within the relationship (see Chapter 3).

In addition to her seminal work detailing the nurse–patient relationship, Peplau developed a nursing model of anxiety. She defined anxiety as a free-floating feeling of apprehension or dread related to a real or perceived threat to self-integrity. According to Peplau, anxiety can be experienced on four different levels:
- *Mild:* Perceptual field widens, increased awareness, problem solving, motivation
- *Moderate:* Can attend to immediate tasks, difficulty with concentration, can be redirected
- *Severe:* Significantly narrowed perceptual field, difficulty problem solving or completing tasks, difficulty learning
- *Panic:* Closed perceptual field, unable to process environmental stimuli, irrational thinking and behavior, potential for self-harm.

Evidence-Based Practice

Evidence-based nursing practice has evolved as the gold standard of psychiatric treatment. Stuart (2009) defines evidence-based practice as "the conscientious explicit, and judicious use of the best evidence gained from systematic research for the purpose of making informed decisions about the care of individual patients" (p. 58). This evidence, combined with the nurse's clinical expertise, consensus recommendations of psychiatric experts, and knowledge of the patient, provides the strongest basis for achieving effective, efficient treatment outcomes. Chapter 10 covers the topic of evidence-based practice in detail.

PSYCHIATRIC–MENTAL HEALTH NURSING PRACTICE

Definition

Psychiatric–mental health nursing is defined as "a specialized area of nursing practice committed to promoting mental health through the assessment, diagnosis, and treatment of human responses to mental health problems and psychiatric disorders" (American Nurses Association [ANA], 2007, p. 1).

Phenomena of Concern for Psychiatric Nurses

The phenomena of concern for psychiatric–mental health nurses relates actual or potential mental health problems of patients across clinical settings, and includes:

- The promotion and maintenance of optimal mental health and well-being and the prevention of mental illness
- Self-care limitations or impaired functioning related to mental, emotional, and physiological distress
- Deficits in the functioning of significant biological, emotional, and cognitive systems
- Emotional stress or crisis related to illness, pain, disability, and loss
- Self-concept and body image changes, developmental issues, life process changes, and end-of-life issues
- Problems related to emotions such as anxiety, anger, confusion, fear, grief, loneliness, powerlessness, and sadness
- Physical symptoms and altered physiological functioning
- Psychological symptoms that occur with altered physiological functioning
- Alterations in communicating, decision-making, perceiving, symbolizing, and thinking
- Difficulties in relating to others
- Behaviors and mental states that indicate the patient is a danger to self or others, or has a severe disability
- Barriers to treatment related to co-occurring disorders such as alcohol and substance abuse and dependency
- Symptom management, side effects/toxicities associated with self-administered drugs, psychopharmacological intervention, and other features of the treatment regimen
- Interpersonal, environmental circumstances or events; organizational, sociocultural, and spiritual issues that affect the mental and emotional well-being of the individual, family, or community
- Socioeconomic factors such as violence and/or poverty

The term *patient* encompasses individuals, families, groups, communities, and populations. *Client* and *mental health consumer* are other terms used to identify people with mental health issues.

Competencies and Skills of Psychiatric Nurses

Knowledge competencies expected of the basic registered nurse in psychiatric–mental health nursing include a theoretical and applied clinical understanding of:

- ANA psychiatric nursing standards,
- Psychiatric diagnoses (DSM-IV; American Psychological Association, 2000),
- Current psychopharmacologic therapies,
- Current non-pharmacologic therapies, and
- Accepted legal and ethical standards.

Basic psychiatric nursing clinical skill expectations include:

- Interviewing techniques,
- Assessment skills,
- Active listening skills, and
- Ability to establish and maintain therapeutic relationships with patients, families, and the multidisciplinary team.

Advanced practice clinical skills, in addition to those listed above, include:

- Diagnosis and assessment of mental disorders,
- Psychotherapy,
- Pharmacologic management of mental disorders, and
- Consultation skills.

Advanced practice nurses can obtain further training in a specialty focus such as sex therapy, marital or family therapy, or therapy with specific populations such as children or older persons.

DIFFERENTIATED NURSING PRACTICE ROLES: A NEW MODEL OF CARE

The American Association of Colleges of Nursing (AACN, 2008) has developed differentiated practice models to help clarify professional nursing role expectations and clinical skills or competencies for clinical interventions and care at different levels of expertise. Differentiated practice models are distinguished from each other by the level of

- Education,
- Expected clinical skills or competencies,
- Participation in decision-making, and
- Professional certification and licensure.

Depending on the clinical setting, a particular nurse's role, position description, and practice setting may further define type or level of practice, for example, in administration, research, education, or clinical practice.

Basic Psychiatric–Mental Health Nursing Practice

AACN (2008) states that roles for the basic nurse are derived from the discipline of nursing and include:

- Provider of care,
- Designer/manager/coordinator of care, and
- Member of a profession.

The registered nurse who practices psychiatric–mental health nursing at the basic level has demonstrated the skills outlined in the *Scope and Standards of Psychiatric–Mental Health Nursing Practice* (ANA, 2007), and has successfully passed the American Nurses Credentialing Center (ANCC) basic psychiatric–mental health certification exam. Basic nursing practice in the specialized area of psychiatric–mental health nursing includes targeted nursing tasks such as:

- Assessing mental health issues and symptoms of mental disorders
- Using interventions to foster and promote optimal mental health
- Assisting patients in regaining or improving their coping abilities, and with self-care skills and activities
- Maximizing patient strengths and preventing further disability

- Administering and monitoring psychobiological treatment regimens (e.g., prescribed psychopharmacological medications and their therapeutic, side, and adverse effects)
- Assisting, promoting, and monitoring patients in self-care activities
- Case management, counseling, and crisis care
- Health maintenance and health promotion
- Health teaching and psycho-education
- Intake screenings, assessment and evaluation of mental health symptoms, and triage
- Milieu therapy (providing a therapeutic environment)
- Psychiatric rehabilitation

Advanced Practice Psychiatric–Mental Health Nursing

The advanced practice nurse in psychiatric–mental health nursing is distinguished by the depth and complexity of knowledge of theory in practice, substantial master's-level clinical practice experience, and expert competence in performing advanced clinical nursing skills. The advanced practice nurse in psychiatric–mental health nursing (APRN-PMH) is prepared to perform all functions of the basic level psychiatric–mental health nurse. Additionally, because of advanced educational preparation and clinical practice expertise, the APRN-PMH is able to perform complex delivery of mental health care services to patients, including:

- *Clinical supervisory responsibilities:* Providing clinical supervision, peer consultations, and peer supervision is a professional and educative development process for growth.
- *Community interventions:* The APRN-PMH assesses the health needs of populations within the community and designs programs for at-risk populations with attention to cultural, developmental, and environmental factors within the community.
- *Case management activities:* Case management involves coordination of services for patients and families, and represents a collaborative model of advocacy and planning for the highest quality, cost-effective care. Case management activities have allowed chronically mentally ill patients to live successfully in the community.

Specific standards for advanced practice psychiatric nurses include

- *Consultation activities:* Advanced practice nurses are equipped to provide consultation to patients (consultation-liaison), staff, and agencies. Legal consultants provide opinions in court cases. Consultation-liaison activities focus on emotional, developmental, spiritual, behavioral, and cognitive responses of patients in general healthcare arenas such as hospitals, rehabilitation centers, and outpatient facilities.
- *Psychopharmacology interventions:* These interventions include prescribing pharmacological agents used to treat mental disorders and ordering and interpreting diagnostic and laboratory tests. The APRN-PMH seeks optimal patient outcomes, anticipates side effects, and ensures against adverse drug reactions/interactions.
- *Psychotherapy:* Psychotherapy is intended to alleviate emotional distress, assist in reversing or changing negative behavior, and assist in facilitating growth. Brief or long-term therapy is provided (e.g., behavioral therapy, insight therapy, solution-focused therapy, Gestalt therapy, psychoanalytic therapy, play therapy) to individuals, couples, groups, or families.

Advanced Practice Nursing Roles

There are four advanced practice roles in nursing:
- Clinical nurse specialist (CNS)
- Certified nurse practitioner (NP)
- Certified midwife
- Certified registered nurse anesthetist (AACN, 2008)

The first two role categories are relevant to advanced practice psychiatric–mental health nursing.

Psychiatric Clinical Nurse Specialist Role

A clinical nurse specialist (CNS) is an advanced practice nurse with a graduate degree in nursing (earned master's or doctorate) who is state licensed as a clinical nurse specialist, and nationally board certified as a CNS by the American Nurses Credentialing Center. Clinical nurse specialists are clinical experts in the diagnosis and treatment of illness and the delivery of evidence-based nursing interventions. Depending on the state, the CNS may or may not have prescriptive authority for psychotropic medications. CNSs work with other healthcare professionals to advance and improve healthcare outcomes and to provide clinical expertise that can result in systemwide changes to improve programs of care. Clinical nurse specialists can practice autonomously as psychotherapists.

The three domains of CNS practice, known as the three "spheres of influence," are the:
- patient/family,
- nursing personnel, and
- system/network organization.

The three spheres overlap and are interrelated, but each sphere possesses a distinctive focus. In each of the spheres of influence, the primary goal of the CNS is continuous improvement of patient outcomes and nursing care. Within the three domains of CNS practice, Sparacinio (2005) identified seven core competencies:
- *Direct clinical practice* includes expertise in advanced assessment, implementing nursing care, and evaluating outcomes.
- *Expert coaching and guidance* encompasses modeling clinical expertise while helping nurses integrate new evidence into practice. It also means providing education or teaching skills to patients and family.
- *Collaboration* focuses on multidisciplinary team-building.
- *Consultation* involves reviewing alternative approaches and implementing planned change.
- *Research* involves interpreting and using research, evaluating practice, and collaborating in research.
- *Clinical and professional leadership* involves responsibility for innovation and change in the patient care system.
- *Ethical decision-making* involves influence in negotiating moral dilemmas, allocating resources, and directing patient care and access to care.

Psychiatric Nurse Practitioner Role

A certified psychiatric nurse practitioner (NP) is an advanced practice nurse with a graduate degree in nursing (earned master's or doctorate) in the specialty, who is state licensed as a psychiatric nurse practitioner and is nationally board certified as a psychiatric or family psychiatric–mental health nurse practitioner. Currently there are two types of psychiatric nurse practitioners credentialed by the ANCC: adult psychiatric nurse practitioner and family psychiatric nurse practitioner.

Psychiatric nurse practitioners are expected to follow National Organization of Nurse Practitioner Faculties (NONPF) guidelines in providing care to patients as a nurse practitioner. NONPF guidelines for psychiatric nursing practice with associated core competencies for the care of individuals and their families and include:
- Diagnose, treat, and clinically manage acute and chronic mental disorders, including pharmacologic management
- Order and interpret diagnostic lab tests
- Teach patients self-management approaches
- Encourage healthy lifestyles
- Consult with multidisciplinary staff regarding patient assessment and care

Psychiatric nurse practitioners practice in collaboration with physicians with a written collaborative agreement. Standardized procedures specify the clinical circumstances in which physician consultation is necessary. Psychiatric nurse practitioners typically consult with a supervising psychiatrist on complex or treatment-resistant cases. Some psychiatric nurse practitioners hold dual certification in adult or family primary care. They can clinically manage patients with illnesses such as asthma, diabetes, hypertension, and so on, in addition to their mental health issues in primary care settings.

CERTIFICATION

The ANCC validates the registered nurse's skills and knowledge through national certification. Certification helps to advance the profession by ensuring the competence and knowledge base of the practitioner in a nursing specialty. Certification is available at the basic and specialist levels for psychiatric–mental health nursing. Additional certifications may be necessary based on further specialization of practice (e.g., practice in marriage and family therapy, addictions counseling).

Basic Psychiatric–Mental Health Nursing Certification

Registered nurses at the basic level who pass the non–advanced practice specialty exam after meeting certain eligibility requirements and after successfully passing the appropriate specialty exam are awarded the Registered Nurse-Board Certified (RN-BC) credential. Criteria for certification as a Basic in Psychiatric Nursing (which must be completed prior to applying for the certification exam) include

- A current, active RN license;
- Clinical practice for the equivalent of 2 years full time as a registered nurse;
- A minimum of 2,000 clinical practice hours in psychiatric–mental health nursing within the past 3 years; and
- A minimum of 30 continuing education hours in psychiatric–mental health nursing within the past 3 years.

Advanced Practice Mental Health Nursing Certification

Advanced practice certification recognizes expert care in a specialty area of nursing. There are four advanced practice nursing roles: certified registered nurse anesthetists, certified nurse-midwives, clinical nurse specialists, and certified nurse practitioners. The advanced practice clinical specialist and nurse practitioner role certifications are relevant for practicing psychiatric–mental health nurses.

The ANCC credential for the advanced practice role of clinical nurse specialist is CNS-BC. The clinical specialty is noted as a prefix in front of the CNS. The credential PMHCNS-BC (Psychiatric–Mental Health CNS-Board Certified) is used for both child/adolescent and adult clinical specialists.

The ANCC credential for the advanced practice role of nurse practitioner is PMHNP–BC for the adult psychiatric–mental health nurse practitioner, and FPMHNP–BC for the family psychiatric–mental health nurse practitioner.

All requirements for advanced practice certification as either a clinical nurse specialist or nurse practitioner in the clinical specialty must be completed prior to applying for the certification examination. Eligibility requirements for the clinical specialist in psychiatric–mental health nursing include:

- Current, active RN license;
- Master's, post-master's, or doctorate degree from a nationally accredited nursing program offering the clinical specialty; and
- Minimum of 500 clinically supervised hours in the specific specialty role. The graduate psychiatric–mental health nursing specialty program must include course work in:
  - Advanced health assessment
  - Advanced pharmacology
  - Advanced pathophysiology
  - Clinical training in at least two psychotherapeutic treatment modalities.

Academic eligibility requirements for the psychiatric nurse practitioner are similar to those required for the clinical nurse specialist, with specific, evidenced clinical practice training as a psychiatric nurse practitioner. Additionally, NP graduate program courses must include content in health promotion and disease prevention and differential diagnosis and disease management.

Recertification

Advanced practice nurses are required to renew their certification every 5 years. ANCC board-certified professional nurses in psychiatric–mental health must meet specified clinical hour and continuing education requirements to maintain and renew their certification. (These requirements are listed on the ANCC website and recertification application forms.)

The purpose of certification renewal is to provide evidence that the certified nurse has continued to expand his or her professional knowledge to remain competent in the certification specialty. Recertification is required if the advanced practice nurse wishes to continue to use ANCC board-certified nursing credentials and practice as an advanced practice nurse.

REFERENCES

American Association of Colleges of Nursing. (1995). *A model for differentiated nursing practice.* Retrieved February 9, 2009, from http://www.picosearch.com/cgi-bin/ts.pl

American Association of Colleges of Nursing. (2008). *Consensus model for APRN regulation: Licensure, accreditation, certification, and education.* Retrieved February 14, 2009, from http://www.aacn.nche.edu/index.htm

American Nurses Association. (2007). *Psychiatric-mental health nursing: Scope and standards of practice.* Silver Spring, MD: Author.

American Psychological Association. (2000). *Diagnostic and statistical manual of mental disorders* (4th ed., text rev.). Washington, DC: Author.

Arnold, W. K., & Nieswiadomy, R. (1993). Peplau's theory with an emphasis on anxiety. In S. M. Ziegler (Ed.), *Theory-directed nursing practice* (pp. 153–178). New York: Springer.

Beck, A. T. (1976/1979). *Cognitive therapy and the emotional disorders.* New York: Penguin Books.

Bowlby J. (1958). The nature of the child's tie to his mother. *International Journal of Psychoanalysis, 39,* 350–373.

Calgary and Area Child and Family Services Authority. (n.d.). *Developmental stages for children/youth.* Retrieved September 10, 2008, from www.calgaryandareacfsa.gov.ab.ca/crv/pdf/Developmental_Stages_Children-Youth.pdf

Cannon, W. (1939). *The wisdom of the body* (2nd ed.). New York: W. W. Norton & Company.

Corbin, J., & Strauss, A. (2000). Chronic illness trajectory framework. *Journal of Advanced Nursing, 32,* 595–602.

Crowley, V. (2000). *Jung: A journey of transformation: Exploring his life and experiencing his ideas.* Wheaton, IL: Quest Books.

Erikson, E. H. (1963). *Childhood and society* (2nd ed.). New York: W. W. Norton & Company.

Evans, F. B. (1996). *Harry Stack Sullivan: Interpersonal theory and psychotherapy.* London: Routledge.

Fawcett, J. (2005). *Contemporary nursing knowledge: Analysis and evaluation of nursing models and theories* (2nd ed.). Philadelphia: F. A. Davis.

Freud, S. (1949). *An outline of psychoanalysis.* New York: W. W. Norton & Company.

Goodman, R., & Scott, S. (2005). *Child psychiatry* (2nd ed.). Hoboken, NJ: Wiley Blackwell.

Kohlberg, L., Levine, C., & Hewer, A. (1983). *Moral stages: A current formulation and a response to critics.* Basel, NY: Karger.

Marrs, J., & Lowery, L. (2006). Nursing theory and practice: Connecting the dots. *Nursing Science Quarterly, 19,* 44–50.

Maslow, A. H. (1943). A theory of human motivation. *Psychological Review, 50*(4), 370–396.

National Panel for Psychiatric Mental Health NP Competencies. (2003). *Psychiatric-mental health nurse practitioner competencies.* Washington, DC: National Organization of Nurse Practitioner Faculties.

Nursingtheory.net. (2005). *Nursing models.* Retrieved February 10, 2009, from http://www.nursingtheory.net/models.html

Peplau, H. (1988). *Interpersonal relations in nursing.* London: Macmillan.

Piaget, J. (1990). *The child's conception of the world.* New York: Littlefield Adams.

Sparacino, P.S.A. (2005). The clinical nurse specialist. In A.B. Hamric, J.A. Spross, & C.M. Hanson (Eds.), *Advanced practice nursing: An integrative approach* (3rd ed., pp. 415–446). St. Louis, MO: Elsevier.

Stuart, G. (2009). *Principles and practice of psychiatric nursing.* St. Louis, MO: Mosby Elsevier.

Communication and the Nurse–Patient Relationship

Elizabeth Arnold, PhD, RN, PMHCNS-BC

Chapter 3 covers therapeutic communication as the primary strategy that psychiatric nurses use to implement all phases of the nurse–patient relationship in psychiatric–mental health nursing. The chapter includes a discussion of therapeutic communication skills (e.g., interpersonal, active listening, verbal vs. nonverbal communication). Relationship issues related to professional boundaries, patient-centered care, attentiveness to cultural and spiritual variables, and the appropriate use of self-awareness are considered. Written documentation and confidentiality issues also are addressed.

THERAPEUTIC COMMUNICATION SKILLS

Therapeutic communication refers to goal-directed conversations with patients aimed at helping patients sort through difficult issues and take thoughtful actions to improve their mental health and well-being. In the field of psychiatric nursing, communication moves to a deeper level as it becomes a primary therapeutic intervention in helping patients consider new constructive perspectives leading to a more productive and satisfying life.

Communication occurs on many different levels, both conscious and unconscious. Factors influencing therapeutic communication involve:
- Culture, language, and ethnic values

- Perceptions of self and other
- Social class
- Developmental stage
- Intellectual processing abilities and skills
- Education
- Setting
- Relationships
- Choice of words and body language
- Timing
- Setting and presentation

Functional Components

The functional components of the communication process include:
- *Sender:* The person who sends a message verbally and nonverbally.
- *Message:* What is actually said, including its nonverbal complement behaviors. Thus, the message includes voice tone, pitch, and bodily movements. The individuals involved in the communication process determine the meaning of the message.
- *Receiver:* The person for whom the message is intended.
- *Feedback:* The response the listener returns to the speaker. Feedback helps patients become aware of how their behavior is perceived by others and how others are interpreting their actions.
- *Context:* The time, place, and situational circumstances surrounding the communication. People respond to the sum total of communication, taking into account the social context in which it is delivered and received. The context includes the relationship dimension and how the participants are connected to each other, related to authority, attitudes, and roles. Cultural and ethnic differences, age, gender, and social status can influence nonverbal communication and interpersonal distance requirements.
- *Channels of communication:* How the communication is transmitted (e.g., hearing, touch, sight, direct discussion, e-mails, phone conversation; Arnold & Boggs, 2007).

Verbal Communication

Language is the crucial medium through which messages are conveyed verbally and in writing. Conversing with others is a socially learned behavior, influenced by sociocultural values and perspectives. Variations in grammar and dialect can affect the meaning of a verbal message. Words can both denote and connote meaning.
- *Denote:* Provide literal meaning
- *Connote:* Imply or suggest a meaning that may or may not be the same as the literal meaning

Anxiety and loss of cognitive processing skills associated with several mental disorders can mean that messages are not fully understood. Psychiatric patients and patients from different cultures can understand concrete verbal messages in which the literal meaning of words is clear, direct, and easy to understand. Empathy, respect, therapeutic authenticity, and being concrete are important components of every therapeutic conversation.

Nonverbal Communication

Nonverbal signals, transmitted through one or more of the human senses, can include body position, body movements, voice quality, use of space, clothing, and personal mannerisms. Culture influences the meaning attributed to these signals, such that the same nonverbal symbol can convey entirely different messages in different cultures. *Metacommunication* is the term used for the nonverbal aspects of communication, such as gestures, facial expressions, and body movements.

Congruent communication takes place when the words and nonverbal components of a personal message match. Incongruent communication occurs when they contradict each other. *Example:* The nurse looking at her watch and telling the patient, "Tell me what is troubling you, I'm here for you." An incongruent match between the words and nonverbal actions gives the patient a mixed message about the nurse's availability.

The nonverbal elements express the relationship aspects of communication. They allow people to express their inner feelings without words, because they are not as easily controlled. Unfortunately, a nonverbal message is more open to misinterpretation.

- *Paralinguistics:* Vocal cues, such as voice pitch, rhythm, pace of words, inflections, and intonations provide the listener with the emotions behind the words. *Example:* Saying "I will attend to it" with caring vocal cues is likely to be perceived differently than if the same statement is said with sarcasm or an impatient intonation.
- *Body position:* Body position can be closed with crossed legs and/or arms, indicating that the person may feel threatened or is not open to conversation. An open body position consisting of eye contact, sitting in a relaxed manner, and leaning forward is indicative of acceptance and openness to conversation.
- *Kinesics:* Nonverbal communication involving muscle or body movement such as eye contact, facial expression, head nodding, smiling
- *Proxemics:* The amount of physical space and distance needed for comfort in conversations between sender and receiver. Culture is an important variable in determining the amount of distance the patient needs to feel comfortable in a therapeutic interaction.
  - Hall (1966) describes 4 distance zones common to conversation: intimate distance, 12 to 18 inches; personal distance, 18 inches to 4 feet; social distance, from 4 to 12 feet; and public distance, 12 feet or more. Most therapeutic conversations take place within personal space.
- *Touch:* A sympathetic touch can be very comforting to small children, frail older adults, and grieving patients. In such situations, touch can be used to give encouragement or to show emotional support. The use of touch, with the exception of therapeutic touch, is largely contraindicated for use with mentally ill patients, because of the danger of misinterpretation.

Attending Behaviors and Active Listening

Attending behaviors and active listening responses are essential components of effective therapeutic communication, and the primary means of effectively responding to a patient's communication.

Attending behaviors involve eye contact, posture, verbal and nonverbal cues. Smiling, leaning forward, nodding, and using facial expression to demonstrate full attention are examples of facilitative, attending behaviors. Sometimes referred to *presence*, attending behaviors demonstrate the nurse's full involvement in "being with" the patient in a mutually interactive relationship.

According to Egan (2002), attending behaviors include
- Open, relaxed, attentive posture
- Facing and leaning slightly towards the patient
- Maintaining appropriate eye contact
- Respecting the interpersonal space of the patient—at least 18 inches
- Removing all unnecessary distractions

Active Listening Response Strategies

Active listening is an interactive, reflective process in which the nurse actively focuses on what a patient is saying with an open attitude and uses a structured form of responses to fully understand the meaning of a communication.

Incorporating attending behaviors and active listening responses ensures mutual understanding of the communication. The nurse responds to the patient in such a way that the patient feels heard and understood. In addition to receiving the patient's message, the nurse examines his or her personal reaction to it, and asks for clarification or validation that the message received is the one the speaker intended. Nurses use nonverbal responses (eye contact, relaxed posture, gestures, leaning forward, facing the person) to display full attention.

In a therapeutic conversation, the patient should do more of the talking than the nurse. The nurse listens for *themes*, representing recurrent patterns or underlying central issues or problems requiring therapeutic intervention. Themes are usually expressed frequently during the course of the interaction.

In addition to conveying interest and acceptance through attending behaviors identified above, the nurse incorporates listening responses to further enhance the depth and breadth of relevant information. These include
- *Broad opening questions:* Questions that cannot be answered with a simple yes or no. Broad, open-ended questions should be neutral so that the patient can set the direction of the conversation. *Example:* "Can you give me a picture of what a typical day would be like for you? Can you tell me what it (this experience) was like for you?
- *Closed questions:* Require a one-word or specific answer; can be used to narrow the topic of discussion or get specific information, but they should be used sparingly.
- *Minimum encouragers:* Offer encouragement with a general minimum verbal lead, which encourages the patient to go into more detail. *Example:* Nodding or saying "uh-huh," "I see," or "go on."
- *Restatement:* Repeating the basic ideas or main thought in the communication by using the patient's own words. Usually only part of the statement is repeated. *Example:* Using opening phrases such as "If I understand you correctly..." or "So what you're saying is...," restate the core part of the patient's message. Restatement should be used sparingly.

- *Paraphrasing*: Recapping the core content components of a patient's message in your own words. The paraphrased message usually is shorter than the original message, and focuses on the *content* of the message. *Example*: Patient: "I am angry with my doctor; it just isn't right that I can't get my privileges." Nurse: "You believe your doctor shouldn't have done this."
- *Reflecting*: In a reflection response, the focus is on the feeling, rather than the content, of the communication. Expressing your perception of the patient's *feelings* in the communication is usually based on a combination of the patient's words, tone, and body language. Timing and respect for cultural differences are important when using reflection responses. *Example*: Patient: "I can't stand how dependent I am on my wife for her approval." Nurse: "It sounds like you feel frustrated by your level of dependence right now. Is that what you are feeling?"
- *Focusing*: Focusing responses are used to help patients examine relevant parts of their communication, usually related to treatment outcomes. A focused question asks the patient for more information about the central issues presented by the patient. It is different from a closed question in that it allows the patient a broader way of responding. *Example*: "I wonder if you could tell me more about how your illness is affecting your relationship with your wife and children."
- *Clarification*: A listening response that signals the listener's need to understand the speaker's situation more fully. It is a way to check perceptions and indicates to the speaker that what he or she is saying is important. *Example*: Patient: "Jerry isn't honest with me. He promises me he will change, but it never lasts more than a few weeks." Nurse: "Marta, I'd like to understand better. Can you give me an example of what you mean by Jerry's being dishonest when he promises to do something, and then doesn't do it?" In addition to asking the patient to provide clarification, the nurse also uses consensual validation as a clarification strategy. *Example*: "It sounds as if Jerry's failure to follow through is very discouraging to you."
- *Empathizing*: An empathizing response verbally acknowledges the patient's emotional state or frame of reference in ways that demonstrate to the speaker that the nurse fully understands and can relate to the patient's situation. Empathy requires that the nurse put her- or himself in the patient's position with compassion and insight without losing the same self. Empathy can also be transmitted nonverbally through tone of voice, authenticity, and congruence among your words, body language, and the attending behaviors described above. *Example*: "I can see how difficult this conversation is for you."
- *Silence*: Appropriately timed silence can be an effective listening response, particularly following expression of an important idea or feeling. The speaker can get significant thoughts together and/or correct a response as he or she reflects inwardly about it. Silence only should be used as a timely pause in relation to a significant communication. Lengthy silence can be awkward and uncomfortable.
- *Summarization*: This strategy is useful either at the end of the session or when the communication is moving to another topic. Effective summaries restate the most important points already covered. They also help the nurse and patient check and refine perceptions about what has been discussed, and in some cases point out areas that need further exploration.

Other helpful communication strategies include
- *Sharing observations*: Nurses share their observations regarding the patient's behavior as a way to help the patient understand his or her emotions. For example: "Your hands are shaking." "You seem upset."

- *Verbalizing implied thoughts and feelings:* The nurse voices what the patient seems to have implied. *Example:* Patient: "It's a waste of time doing these exercises." Nurse: "You feel that they aren't benefiting you?"
- *Giving information:* As nurses, we educate and provide specific information. Studies have shown that a major cause of anxiety in hospitalized patients is lack of information or misconceptions about their condition, treatment, or hospital routine. Education is a primary nursing function. Providing facts in an objective manner allows the patient to accept or reject them. It is up to individual patients how and to what extent they will use the information.
- *Giving feedback:* Feedback is an essential component of therapeutic communication. Effective feedback should be
  - Immediate, honest, reflective, constructive, and nonjudgmental
  - Focused on the behavior, not the person or emotion
  - Focused only on behaviors, which can be changed
  - Given in a private setting

BARRIERS TO EFFECTIVE COMMUNICATION

Defensive patient communication occurs when a person perceives or anticipates a threat as part of a conversation. As a person becomes defensive, he or she is less able to accurately perceive the true motives or intent of a communication. Freud introduced the concept of ego defense mechanism as a form of defensive communication that patients use when they perceive a threat to self-integrity.

Ego Defense Mechanisms

Ego defense mechanisms are defined as unconscious methods that people use to protect themselves from consciousness of a threat to self. By distorting the meaning of the original threat, the defense mechanism makes it less anxiety-provoking to the person. The use of a defense mechanism distances the person from a full awareness of unpleasant thoughts, feelings, desires, or impulses. Common defense mechanisms include:

- *Denial:* Acting as though a painful circumstance, situation, feeling, or thought doesn't exist. *Example:* Denying that you are an alcoholic despite its negative impact on your marital relationship.
- *Rationalization:* Supplying a logical reason for a behavior to justify it. *Example:* Contending that the only reason you have two martinis for lunch every day is because you are a salesman, and drinking at lunch is expected.
- *Displacement:* Directing unacceptable feelings, impulses, or thoughts onto a safer, less threatening target. *Example:* Being angry at your boss but not verbalizing it, coming home and getting angry at your wife for the way she handles the house.
- *Regression:* Reversion to an earlier stage of development. *Example:* Toddler who reverts to wanting a bottle or pacifier and soils his pants when his baby brother is born.
- *Repression:* An unconscious forgetting, usually of a traumatic event or feeling. *Example:* Forgetting being sexually abused as a child.

- *Reaction formation:* Taking the opposite position to an unacceptable belief. *Example:* A person with strong addictive impulses leads a crusade against addiction.
- *Projection:* Attribution of one's shameful or undesired impulses, thoughts, or feelings onto another. *Example:* An angry person accuses her partner of being hostile.
- *Suppression:* The conscious dismissing of an unacceptable idea, desire, painful memory, and so on, from the mind. Suppression can be a positive defense mechanism, used to eliminate negative thinking. *Example:* A person is thinking about the possibility of a promotion so much it is compromising his work. He decides not to think about it and just go with the flow of his present job in the best way possible.
- *Sublimation:* The channeling of unacceptable impulses into more acceptable outcomes. *Example:* A person with very aggressive tendencies becomes a butcher.
- *Undoing:* The person tries to take back behavior, feelings, or thoughts that are unacceptable to him or her by partially negating a previous communication or action. *Example:* When asked for a recommendation, a person makes derogatory remarks about a friend to her employer, and then praises the good work her friend is doing for the company in the same interaction.

Non-Therapeutic Communication Strategies

- *Giving false reassurance:* Statements such as: "You're doing just fine" minimize the patient's concerns. Don't offer false reassurance. Share your observations instead and let the patient interpret their meaning.
- *Giving advice:* Direct advice imposes the nurse's own opinions and solutions on the patient and is inappropriate. Clarify and use other communication techniques to help patients come to their own solutions.
- *Making stereotypical comments:* Drawing a conclusion about a person based on general knowledge of ethnicity, gender, or social status rather than considering each person's attributes. Regard each individual as a unique human being.
- *Changing the subject:* Arbitrarily changing the subject so the nurse directs the course of the conversation can make the patient feel unimportant and abandoned. Sometimes it occurs when the nurse is uncomfortable with the topic. Identify the source of your discomfort and work it through; then you will be able to use silence and really listen.
- *Moralizing or being judgmental:* Imposition of the nurse's values onto the patient implies that the nurse is entitled to make a value judgment regarding the patient's feelings or behavior. Keep an open mind and recognize that all behavior has meaning even if you don't understand it.
- *Minimizing or belittling the patient's feelings:* Statements such as "I know just how you feel" or "Everyone gets depressed sometimes" deny the importance of the patient's feelings and perceptions as unique. Each individual reacts and responds differently. This approach shifts the focus from the patient to the nurse ("I know...") or others ("Everyone gets..."). Acknowledge the patient's feeling or information-sharing instead.
- *Disagreeing with the patient:* "You're wrong." "That's not true." Although this can be used appropriately as a reality check, it can indicate that what the patient said has not been accepted. Use giving information or tentative reflective questions instead.
- *Tangential or irrelevant comment:* Trite sayings such as "You have a lot to be grateful for" or "Isn't it a beautiful day?" keep the conversation at a superficial level. Try starting with a broad opening statement instead.

PATIENTS WITH SPECIAL COMMUNICATION NEEDS

Adapting Communication Style to Enhance Understanding

Effective communication requires that psychiatric nurses modify their communication style to accommodate the specialized needs of their clients. This can include sensory alterations (visual, hearing impaired), speaking a different language, literacy level, developmental stage, or cognitive status (Potter & Perry, 2009). The following are communication modifications.

Patients With Visual Impairments
- Make sure the patient has appropriate glasses or contacts
- Use large print for visual instructions
- Use a normal tone and pace for conversation
- Orient the patient to the area, describing significant elements and boundaries
- Identify yourself when entering the patient's space
- Look directly at the patient when speaking

Patients With Hearing Impairments
- Minimize background noise
- Always face the patient when speaking
- Speak slowly, in a normal tone; the tone can be slightly raised if the person is not completely deaf (do not shout)
- If the patient has a hearing aid, make sure the patient is wearing it, and that it is turned on
- Rephrase, rather than repeat if the communication is not understood

Patients With Cognitive Impairments
- Assess the patient's ability to communicate
- Make adaptations with simpler, concrete words if needed
- Speak slowly and clearly
- Repeat or rephrase questions if the patient looks puzzled
- Use simple questions and allow extra time for response
- Look at and speak directly to the patient when speaking

Patients With English as a Second Language
- Avoid using family members as interpreters
- Speak slowly and clearly
- Use simple language and pause between sentences
- Validate the patient's understanding by asking for frequent brief summaries
- Look at the patient when speaking, even when using an interpreter
- Make allowances for differences in idioms, personal space, ritual, expression of emotions, parent-child interactions, customs, and so on
- Allow extra time for the interview

Patients From a Different Culture
Communication is always to some degree culture-bound, and should be considered a critical component in professional therapeutic relationships. Since people respond to situations and experiences based on their worldview and personal values, it is important for nurses to be aware

of personal cultural orientations in therapeutic conversations with patients from different ethnic groups. Madeleine Leininger's Theory of Transcultural Nursing (Sunrise model) offers a good review of the areas of culturally sensitive beliefs, values, and practices, which nurses need to incorporate as background information in therapeutic conversations with ethnically diverse patients.

At the same time, each individual patient is different. There is more variation in values within a culture than between cultures. (See Chapter 5 for terminology related to cultural diversity and competence.) Asking patients directly about cultural interpretations of mental illness and treatment is as important as having a basic cultural knowledge of ethnic values and behaviors. Incorporating ethnic values and paying attention to the cultural concerns of patients from different cultures are essential steps that increase understanding and make conversations go more smoothly. Other relevant communication strategies can include:

- Keeping questions simple, concrete, and specific
- Choosing unambiguous words with single, rather than connotative, meanings
- Respecting differences in the amount of interpersonal space and meaning of body language among different cultural groups
- Asking only one question at a time
- Using multiple methods to convey information (e.g., pictures, physical cues)
- Having the patient repeat back, in his or her own words, key ideas and teaching content

Communicating About Spiritual Matters

Spirituality is defined as a person's values and beliefs about his or her place in the universe and the presence of a higher power in matters of life, health, and death. A person's spiritual orientation is often an important way for patients to make sense of their illness and the things that are happening to them as a result. Spiritual worldviews, including atheism and agnosticism, develop over time. A person's spiritual orientation may or may not be tied to a defined religious framework. Nurses need to be aware of, objective, and nonjudgmental about a patient's religious and spiritual beliefs.

Current Joint Commission standards mandate assessment of a patient's spiritual needs as part of the overall health assessment. The spiritual needs assessment should include the patient's denomination, beliefs, and spiritual practices that are important to the patient, and information should be documented in the patient's plan of care. On its website, The Joint Commission includes sample questions to ask patients and their families about spiritual needs (The Joint Commission, 2008). The purpose of doing a spiritual assessment is to determine the most appropriate actions needed to address these issues. Assessment data with related actions must be documented in the patient's care plan.

Although religious content can reflect symptomatology in individuals with mental illness, for many patients, spirituality is like an island in a stormy sea. Nurses need to be able to distinguish between pathologic religiosity and spiritual dependence on a higher power. Many patients with mental illness experience loneliness and isolation. Believing that a personal god is always with you can be comforting and strengthening. Spirituality gives many patients a measured sense of control over their illness and has been associated with positive outcomes, such as a decrease in mental symptoms (Carson & Koenig, 2008).

The language of faith is often learned prior to the development of a mental illness. Some patients find spirituality painful because they view their illness as a punishment from God, or a betrayal of their adherence to religious beliefs. For these patients, helping them to correct or decrease the impact of painful feelings associated with negative spiritual images can be a useful intervention. Cognitive strategies can help these patients question the validity of their current thinking, and shift their negative spiritual images to more productive explanations of the role of a higher power in their lives.

Strategies When the Patient Is Aggressive or Uncooperative

Aggressiveness in mental health settings has many possible causes, and can be exacerbated by comorbid substance abuse, impulsiveness, hallucinations (particularly command hallucinations), dementia, or antisocial personality traits. Patients with mental retardation can become violent when exposed to chaotic circumstances or overcrowding. Delirium and other forms of severe brain dysfunction caused by medical or psychiatric disorders can also stimulate aggressive episodes. Basically, any situation in which a patient feels loss of control can stimulate anger and potential aggression.

Most patients who are angry, manipulative, or uncooperative are extremely anxious and feel misunderstood. Addressing the deeper-rooted anxiety and validating the patient's feelings can help defuse a tense situation. Other facilitative strategies include expressing caring and empathy: "I can see that you are very upset. How can I help you?"

- Observe for prodromal signs of impending tension (eyes or mouth twitching, pacing, flinging arms, spitting, increased agitation).
- Check for nonverbal messages. Say "I notice that you are wringing your hands and you are pacing down the hallway. Can you tell me what you are feeling?"
- Be aware that the patient's words reflect his or her feelings about a stressful situation and are not directed toward you personally.
- Address the patient by name, and speak in a low, calm voice.
- Assess the environment and the patient for signs of escalating tension. Identify triggers. Remember that aggressive patients may be experiencing intense anxiety and may not be able to explain the cause of their agitation.
- Give the patient extra space; avoid crowding the patient, as this may be misinterpreted as aggression or a desire to control.
- Use "I" statements, with concrete comments. *Example:* "I am concerned about your safety and the safety of others right now, as you are swearing and yelling loudly. I need for you to quiet down so we can figure this out."
- Own your own feelings.
- Criticize the behavior, not the individual: "I want you to know that I care about your and others' health on this unit. However, your behavior of yelling and stomping around the unit is not acceptable."
- Positive stroking: Find something genuinely positive to say, such as "I admire how you were able to calm down after your father came to visit. I am confident you can calm down today, as well."
- Point out what is in it for the patient: "I really can't help you, unless we can talk about _____ in a calmer way."

- Balancing message: "I know that what you are going through is very difficult for you. However, I know that you have the strength within you to cope in a manner that will help you in the long run."
- Summon extra help for a "show of force" or a "show of concern." Do not try to subdue an aggressive patient by yourself; use a planned team approach.

Communicating in Conflict Situations

Conflicts are inevitable, and working through them can make a relationship stronger. Encourage collaboration, which stimulates cooperation.
- Both parties state their problem.
  - Use "I" statements.
  - Indicate a willingness to help resolve the problem.
  - Stick to the topic at hand.
- Hear the other person's point of view.
  - Acknowledge the patient's anger.
  - Don't interrupt unless patient is repeating him- or herself, then rephrase what was said.
- Acknowledge the patient's viewpoint.
  - Ask clarifying questions.
  - Use silence.
  - Rehearse.
- Look for areas of agreement.
  - Point out mutual interests.
  - Make an optimistic statement.
- Request behavior changes only.
- Help patients help themselves develop realistic solutions.
- Whenever possible, focus on solutions that satisfy the needs of both parties.

THERAPEUTIC RELATIONSHIPS

Definition

Hildegard Peplau defined the therapeutic relationship in psychiatric nursing as a professional, patient-centered alliance in which a qualified nurse joins with a patient experiencing a mental healthcare need to meet health-related treatment goals. Treatment outcomes relate to improving a patient's mental health and well-being (Peplau, 1997).

Nursing Role

Heavily influenced by Harry Stack Sullivan's interpersonal framework, Peplau conceptualized the nurse's role in a therapeutic relationship as that of *participant observer*. In a therapeutic alliance with a patient, the nurse is an active participant and the primary tool psychiatric nurses use is the self. As participants in the nurse–patient relationship, nurses share a partnership with their patients, focused on the patient's recovery. They play key roles in helping patients move in the direction of health and well-being. These roles include:

- *Stranger:* Meeting and accepting the patient as a unique person.
- *Counselor:* Counseling patients related to current problems.
- *Healthcare resource person:* Interpreting the treatment plan to the patient, and helping him or her access relevant treatment resources.
- *Teacher:* Providing relevant information and helping the patient learn.
- *Leader:* Mediating, acting as a safety agent.

Regardless of which role the nurse assumes when providing care for patients, genuineness, respect, concreteness, and empathy should be basic features in every therapeutic conversation.

As observers, nurses consistently scrutinize the patient's behavior, their own behaviors, and the nature of nurse–patient exchanges for interpersonal connections and disconnects.

Self-Awareness

Peplau (1997) noted that nurses must observe their own behavior, as well as the patient's, with "unflinching self-scrutiny and total honesty in assessment of their behavior in interactions with patients." Effective psychiatric nurses have a good sense of self-awareness about themselves— their strengths, weaknesses, actions, reactions, motivations, and personal beliefs. Self-awareness allows the nurse to act authentically and to remain centered, even in complicated situations. In addition to self-reflection, nurses can increase their professional self-awareness of issues affecting the nurse–patient relationship through regular peer supervision. Seeking consultation with expert nurses when confronted with transference or countertransference issues that threaten the integrity of the nurse–patient relationship is also useful.

The Johari Window (Figure 3–1) provides a graphic model used to develop self-awareness. Although no one has total access to his or her personality, it is possible through communication with others to know oneself and be known by others. When a person expands the data in one quadrant, the other three reduce in size. The larger quadrant 1 is, the greater the self-awareness. The best way to decrease the size of quadrant 2 is to listen attentively to the feedback of others about their perceptions of you. Self-disclosure is a helpful way to decrease the size of quadrant 3 (Stuart, 2009).

Figure 3–1. Johari Window

1 Known to Self and Others	2 Known Only to Others
3 Known Only to Self	4 Known Neither to Self nor to Others

Note. Originally developed by Luft, J., & Ingham, H. (1955). The Johari window: A graphic model of interpersonal awareness. Proceedings of the western training laboratory in group development. Los Angeles: UCLA.

Phases of the Therapeutic Relationship

Peplau identified distinct sequential phases of the therapeutic relationship as part of her interpersonal theory: the orientation, working, and termination phases. The phases are equally applicable in inpatient and outpatient settings. Each phase has specific therapeutic tasks or goals.

- The *orientation phase* sets the stage for the relationship. Nursing tasks include:
  - Developing a therapeutic alliance
  - Establishing therapeutic boundaries related to the structure of the relationship; confidentiality
  - Mutually defining the therapeutic contract (time, place, duration of each meeting, and length of relationship)
  - Building trust and rapport
  - Assessing patient needs, strengths, and coping strategies
  - Identifying nursing diagnoses based on assessment data
  - Specifying treatment outcomes directly related to nursing diagnoses and initial treatment objectives
- *Working phase* is the phase in which most of the therapeutic work takes place. Peplau divided this phase into two sub-phases: an identification phase and an exploitive phase. In the identification phase, the nurse and patient collaborate in looking at the assessment data, clarify expectations, and develop a realistic plan of care. The exploitive component of the working phase can be more intense, focusing on:
  - Teaching patients new skills
  - Implementing a realistic plan of action related to identified therapeutic goals
  - Evaluating and modifying realistic goals, with related plans of action, to achieve identified treatment outcomes
- *Termination phase.* No new work is begun in the termination phase. The termination of the therapeutic relationship occurs when mutually agreed-upon therapeutic goals are achieved, or the patient is discharged or transferred to another facility. Tasks focus on:
  - Reviewing accomplishments and patient progress toward therapeutic goals
  - Exploring the need for referrals post-discharge
  - Establishing plans for long-term post-discharge functioning
  - Moving towards closure of the relationship

Ideally, the patient will demonstrate greater emotional stability and more effective coping skills as treatment outcomes resulting from effective therapeutic relationships. Some patients demonstrate temporary regressive behaviors, hostility, or sadness that the relationship is ending.

Factors that enhance the effectiveness of a therapeutic relationship include consistency, pacing, encouraging active patient collaboration, and willingness to listen. Establishing and maintaining authentic, flexible professional boundaries in all phases of the therapeutic relationship helps protect the integrity of nurse–patient interaction (Varcolis, Carson, & Shoemaker, 2006).

Professional Boundaries

Professional boundaries make the nurse–patient relationship safe. They clarify the nurse's role in the relationship and distinguish this relationship as a professional alliance distinct from the patient's personal relationships. Therapeutic boundaries are the invisible interpersonal limits surrounding professional relationships that specify time, proximity, and distance between nurse and patient; informed consent; level of relationship; nontreatment meetings; clothing; language; gift-giving; touch; and professional self-disclosure. The most grievous boundary violation is that of a sexual nature, which is never permitted under any circumstance.

The nurse, not the patient, is responsible for establishing and maintaining the boundaries in the therapeutic nurse–patient relationship. Boundary violations occur any time a professional nurse enters into a social, financial, or personal relationship with a patient. Boundary crossings are lesser transgressions that can involve role, time, place, or financial boundaries. They generally fall in the realm of structuring the relationship, self-disclosure, gift-giving, touch, involvement in the patient's life outside of treatment, and involvement in dual relationships. Warning signs of boundary violations related to the structure of the relationship can include

- Feeling that you understand the patient's problems better than other members of the healthcare team
- Giving certain patients extra time or attention
- Spending off-duty time with patients
- Giving patients personal contact information
- Failing to set limits with patients
- Giving patients money to buy snacks

Self-disclosure is a deliberate, reflective interpersonal strategy in which the nurse shares personal information for the purpose of enhancing the therapeutic relationship. When self-disclosure is brief, focused, and relevant to the goals of the relationship, it can be useful to the therapeutic relationship. It strengthens the bond between nurse and patient, and reassures patients that their problems are not unique. Self-disclosure should be used judiciously and sparingly, and only to meet an identifiable therapeutic patient need. Without a direct connection to meeting a patient's therapeutic need, self-disclosure by the nurse is ill-advised.

Giving or accepting gifts from patients: Nurses should refrain from giving or accepting gifts unless it is an appropriate token gift that meets an identified therapeutic need and doesn't change the therapeutic dynamics of the relationship.
Touch and physical contact: Nurses should consider the possible meaning of touch and physical contact with mentally ill patients. While limited touch may be helpful with dementia patients, children, or a grieving patient, in general it should be avoided.
Involvement in the patient's personal life: Nurses should not interfere in a patient's personal life. Meeting with patients outside of treatment sessions is not appropriate, and can sabotage the therapeutic work.
Dual relationships: Co-existing relationships can undermine the therapeutic judgment and objectivity needed for therapeutic care. Examples include providing professional nursing care to a friend, engaging in business relationships with patients, and establishing outside relationships or friendships with patients.

Therapeutic Impasses

The most common types of therapeutic impasses in nurse–patient relationships include resistance, transference, countertransference, and boundary violations.

- *Resistance* refers to the patient's reluctance to reveal relevant information about his or her experience, feelings, or level of symptoms. It is an unconscious process that may reflect the patient's unwillingness to change, or fear of change. Resistance is most likely to occur in the working phase, because this is the problem-solving phase associated with making therapeutic changes.
- *Transference* is the process whereby a patient inappropriately transfers attitudes and emotional reactions originally linked with significant people in the past onto current relationships.
  - *Splitting* occurs when a patient displays a positive dependent transference toward one staff member while demeaning the competence of other staff members.
- *Countertransference* is the nurse's unconscious displacement of feelings associated with past relationships onto the current relationship with a patient. Countertransference feelings are evidenced when the nurse feels very positive or negative feelings toward a patient that are not justified.

The key to handling a therapeutic impasse in the nurse–patient relationship is to acknowledge its existence, explore its role in stalling the relationship, and clarify relationship goals. If the nurse is experiencing countertransference, seeking supervision from an expert nurse is advised.

WRITTEN COMMUNICATION AND DOCUMENTATION OF CARE

Charting in the Patient's Record

Written documentation of the patient assessment, treatment, patient response, and progress is an important component of the communication process in psychiatric–mental health nursing. Documentation refers to the written legal recording of patient care. Unless care is documented in the patient's record, from a legal perspective it is as though it wasn't done. The patient's medical record is often presented in court as evidence of assessment and treatment. In many instances, the written medical record is the sole informant about the care given to patients.

Written communication/documentation includes objective and subjective assessment data about the patient's condition or mental health issues, interdisciplinary plans and treatment, restrictive measures if employed, treatment plan/outcome documentation, risk-assessment documentation, mental status, occurrence reports, treatment response, etc.

Charted documentation is written in ink with no erasures. If there is a mistake in the documentation, the nurse should cross out the error with one line, insert the corrected information if needed, and initial the change. Charting should be completed after the care is given, not before.

The three most common documentation methods include narrative documentation, SOAP notes (see below), and focus charting. A fourth method, exception charting, is used in some agencies and institutions (Arnold & Boggs, 2007).

- *Narrative documentation* reflects the format of the nursing process. It includes objective and subjective assessment data about the patient's condition or mental health issues, interdisciplinary plans and treatment, restrictive measures if employed, treatment plan/outcome documentation, risk-assessment documentation, mental status, occurrence reports, treatment response, and so on. The data are recorded in sequential order covering a specified time frame. Depending on the facility, flow sheets and checklists can be used to document routine care such as activities of daily living, personal care, vital signs, and so on, as well as standardized observations.

- *Problem-oriented charting (SOAP/SOAPIER)* is a format wherein the nurse lists patient problems in order of priority, followed by the plan, intervention, and evaluation, including any needed changes or revisions. The following headings are used in problem-oriented charting:

  S = Subjective data
  O = Objective data
  A = Assessment data
  P = Plan
  I = Intervention
  E = Evaluation
  R = Revision

Here too, flow charts and checklists are used by many agencies to document routine, ongoing assessments and patient responses. Information recorded on flow sheets or checklists is not repeated in the progress notes.

- *Focus charting* requires the nurse to identify a particular focus based on a careful assessment of individualized patient behaviors or health concerns. The focus can be directly on a particular behavior or concern, such as aggressive or catatonic behavior, or it can reflect a change in a patient's condition or behavior, such as a delirium. It can also reflect a significant event in the patient's treatment, for example, an ECT treatment. With focus charting, the nurse documents should include:
  - Subjective and objective data, supporting the stated focus
  - Actions: Completed nursing interventions related to the nurse's focused assessment
  - Response: Description of the patient's response, and the impact of interventions on patient outcomes

- *Documentation by exception.* Some clinical agencies use documentation by exception. This type of charting assumes that assessment findings, nursing interventions, and clinical outcomes will follow the agency's established written standards of care. Charting by exception assumes that all relevant standards of care have been met with the expected treatment response, unless documented otherwise. The only other exclusion is for medication administration, which must be charted directly.

Clinical Pathways

Many inpatient settings use written clinical pathways to direct and coordinate care for psychiatric patients (Stuart, 2009). Clinical pathways are developed by multidisciplinary team members and are linked to clinical and quality improvement outcomes. They can be organized according to DSM-IV-TR diagnosis, The North American Nursing Diagnosis Association (NANDA) International diagnoses, treatment stages, clinical interventions, or targeted behaviors. The clinical pathway document identifies key clinical processes, with corresponding timelines so that all relevant treatment team members can document their assessments and patient progress on one record of care. In a growing number of clinical settings, the clinical pathway is computerized. Key components of a clinical pathway include:

- Identifying a target population
- Describing the expected outcome of treatment in a measurable, realistic, and patient-centered way
- Specifying treatment strategies, variances, and goal achievement
- Documenting patient care activities, variances, and goal achievement (Stuart, 2009, p. 62)

Clinical Algorithms

Clinical algorithms represent a sequential flowchart related to possible treatment options, use of medications, and progress assessment. The chart is presented as a set of guidelines, which "make explicit the art of diagnostic reasoning" (Stuart, 2009, p. 62). Each algorithm uses a decision tree format featuring decision points requiring a yes or no response, or range of lab values. This offers the advantage of providing clinicians with evidence-based standards for sound clinical practice in a timely manner. Clinical algorithms provide a standardized way to compare a patient's actual progress with expected progress guidelines. Computerized clinical algorithms are increasingly being used in mental health settings to improve clinical decision making.

Use of Technology in Documentation

More and more clinical agencies and hospitals are using electronic health records as the primary form of documentation. If this is the case, all of the principles identified above for charting formats, access, storage, and retrieval of patient information are identical to those that govern paper-based documentation. Nurses must ensure the complete integrity of the electronic record.

Most agencies have strict policies for the use of electronic documentation. Of particular importance is the need to carefully protect personal identification numbers or passwords. Passwords should not be shared or revealed to others. They should not be easily decipherable. Nurses should always log off when leaving a terminal or otherwise not using the system, and protect patient information displayed on monitors while using the system.

REFERENCES

Adubato, S. (2004). Making the communication connection. *Nursing Management, 35*(9), 33–35.

Arnold, E., & Boggs, K. (2007). *Interpersonal relationships in nursing* (5th ed.). Philadelphia: Elsevier.

Boyd, M. A. (2007). *Psychiatric nursing: Contemporary practice* (4th ed.). Philadelphia: Lippincott Williams & Wilkins.

Carson, V., & Koenig H. (Eds.). (2008). *Spiritual dimensions of nursing practice.* West Conshohocken, PA: Templeton Foundation Press.

Egan, G. (2002). *The skilled helper: A problem management and opportunity development approach to helping* (7th ed.). Pacific Grove, CA: Brooks/Cole.

Gutheil, T., & Gabbarad, G. (1993). The concept of boundaries in clinical practice: Theoretical and risk management dimensions. *American Journal of Psychiatry, 150,* 188–196.

Hall, E. T. (1966). *The hidden dimension.* New York: Doubleday

Institute of Medicine Committee on Quality of Health Care in America. (2001). *Crossing the quality chasm: A new health system for the 21st century.* Washington, DC: Author.

The Joint Commission. (2008). *Spiritual assessment.* Retrieved February 1, 2009, from http://www. jointcommission.org/AccreditationPrograms/Hospitals/Standards/09_FAQs/PC/Spiritual_ Assessment.htm

Luft, J., & Ingham, H. (1955). The Johari window: A graphic model of interpersonal awareness. *Proceedings of the western training laboratory in group development.* Los Angeles: UCLA.

Newman, C. (2005). Too close for comfort: Defining boundary issues in the professional-client relationship. *Rehabilitation & Community Care Medicine, Spring,* 7–9.

Peplau, H. E. (1991). *Interpersonal relations in nursing: A conceptual frame of reference for psychodynamic nursing.* New York: Springer.

Peplau, H. E. (1997). Peplau's theory of interpersonal relations. *Nursing Science Quarterly, 10*(4), 162–167.

Potter P., & Perry, A. (2009). *Fundamentals of nursing* (7th ed.). St. Louis, MO: Mosby Elsevier.

Peterneij-Taylor, C. A., & Yonge, O. (2003). Exploring boundaries in the nurse client relationship: Professional roles and responsibilities. *Perspectives in Psychiatric Care, 39*(2), 55–66.

Smith, L. L., Taylor, B. B., Keys, A. T., & Gornto, S. B. (1997). Nurse–patient boundaries: Crossing the line. *American Journal of Nursing, 97*(12), 26–32.

Stuart, G. (2009). *Principles and practice of psychiatric nursing* (9th ed.). St. Louis, MO: Elsevier Mosby.

Varcolis, E. M., Carson, V. B., & Shoemaker, N. (2006). *Foundations of psychiatric mental health nursing: A clinical approach* (5th ed.). St. Louis, MO: Saunders/Elsevier.

4

Evidence-Based Psychiatric Nursing Practice

Karan Kverno, PhD, PMHNP-BC, PMHCNS-BC

The essentials of psychiatric–mental health nursing, its activities and accountabilities, and distinctions between the basic and advanced levels of practice, are articulated in the *Psychiatric-Mental Health: Scope and Standards of Practice* (American Nurses Association [ANA], 2007). Psychiatric–mental health nursing is defined as "a specialized area of nursing practice committed to promoting mental health through the assessment, diagnosis, and treatment of human responses to mental health problems and psychiatric disorders" (p. 14). This chapter presents an overview of the nursing process for the psychiatric–mental health nurse.

The steps of the nursing process:
1. Assessment
2. Diagnosis
3. Outcome identification
4. Planning
5. Implementation
6. Evaluation

ASSESSMENT

The assessment includes the systematic and continuous collection of data about the health status of the patient. The primary sources of the data are the patient interview, direct observation, labs, and other test results. Secondary sources may include family members, members of the healthcare team, or other involved individuals (e.g., school reports). The following types of data are collected:

- Biographical information
- Reason for seeking health care
- Current medical and psychosocial status
  - Mental status exam
  - Motivation, coping responses
  - Relationships, spiritual beliefs, and values
  - Strengths and competencies
  - Ability to remain safe and refrain from harming others
  - Risk factors: falls, pain, violence, suicidal (S/I) or homicidal (H/I) ideation
- Psychiatric and medical history
  - Growth and development
  - Previous psychiatric episodes and treatments
  - Previous medical symptoms or illnesses and their treatments
- Allergies, medications, and reactions
- History of substance use
- Family, sociocultural, and occupational history
- Review of systems and general functioning
- Vital signs and lab values

Cultural Sensitivity

Culture is an important context within which to view an individual or family. A brief cultural assessment would include identifying:

- How the person identifies him- or herself
- Degree of acculturation/immigration
- Affinity of the person to the native culture or to the host culture
- Language use, abilities, and preferences
- Cultural interpretations of functional levels

The Mental Status Exam

The Mental Statuse Exam (MSE) is a *subjective* report of the patient's current mental state as observed by the nurse. Assessment of mental status is a continuous part of the nursing process. When MSE findings are reported, they consist of what the nurse observed *at the time* of the interaction: not before and not after. Screening and assessment tools, such as the Mini-Mental Status Exam (Folstein, Folstein, & McHugh, 1975) provide *objective* indicators of current mental status. Box 4–1 describes the components of the MSE.

Box 4-1. Components of the Mental Status Exam

Appearance and Behavior

- Overall appearance related to age, culture
- Hygiene and grooming
- Style, appropriateness of clothing to age, weather, occasion
- Posture and mannerisms
- General behavior (e.g., impulsivity, passive, hostile, fearful)
- Motor behavior (e.g., pacing, lethargic, catatonic)
- Attitude toward clinician and willingness to cooperate.

Mood and Affect

- Mood: Internal feelings that influence behavior (e.g., depressed, suspicious, elated, euthymic)
- Affect: Emotional expression variation; found in face, voice, use of body movements (e.g., flat, guarded, inappropriate, blunted, restricted, labile)

Thought Processes

- Continuity and organization of ideas
  - Problems with word-finding
  - Processing of abstract ideas
  - Blocking, unexpected thought stoppage
- Flow and rhythm: Slowed or racing thoughts
- Logical coherency of ideas
- Amount: Excessive speech or poverty of speech
- Language or meaning deficits

Processing Deficits

- Clanging: Choice of words based on similar sounds, not associated ideas
- Echolalia: Repetition of other people's words or phrases
- Neologisms: Creation of new words that don't make sense
- Word salad: Disorganized, senseless progression of words
- Perseveration: Tedious repetition of the same words or ideas regardless of stimuli
- Flight of ideas: Ideas are not logically connected, abrupt changes in topic
- Loose associations: Limited or no logical progression between words or ideas
  - Circumstantial: Excessive and unnecessary detail, eventually answering the question
  - Tangential: Never returns to the point or answers the question
- Thought-blocking: Interruption or delay in thought processing, not related to lack of concentration, distraction, or anxiety

Evaluation of Thought Content

- Suicide: Plan, opportunity, means?
- Homicide: Victim, realistic plan?
- Delusions: Fixed, false beliefs
- Phobias: Intense, unreasonable fears
- Obsessions: Intrusive, repetitious

Continued

Box 4-1. Components of the Mental Status Exam (cont.)

Delusional Thinking

- Delusions: False beliefs that cannot be dislodged by logic or contradictory evidence; not congruent with normative culture or religious beliefs
  - Of reference: Other people's thoughts, words, or actions refer to self
  - Persecution: Other people have malevolent intentions toward self, or are conspiring against the person
  - Religious: Unrealistic special relationship with God
  - Nihilistic: Destruction of self, world, or body part
  - Grandiose: Special, gifted, powerful, or important without factual support

Perception

- Depersonalization: Feeling detached or as if one is an outside observer of one's mental processes or body
- Illusions: False perceptions
- Déjà vu or flashbacks
- Hallucinations: Differ among the medical and psychiatric disorders
  - Delirium: May be accompanied by visual and/or aural hallucinations
  - Dementia: Visual hallucinations are common with Lewy body dementia
  - Depression with psychotic factors: Mood-congruent (e.g., hearing people whisper criticisms in depression)
  - Seizures or brain injury: Visual, auditory, tactile, gustatory, olfactory
  - Schizophrenia: Generally auditory, may be mood-incongruent (person may seem euthymic but hear command to harm another person [command hallucination]); bizarre hallucinations, such as hearing a conversation between several people, are suggestive of schizophrenia
  - Substance-related intoxication or withdrawal: Any kind; depends on the drug

Sensorium and Cognition

- Memory recall: Immediate, recent, remote
- Orientation to person, time, and place
- Concentration: Serial 7s (keep in mind educational level)
- Abstract thinking
- Disturbances suggest organic dysfunction due to meds, substance abuse, cognitive disorder

Judgment

- Realistic decision-making based on:
  - Current level of knowledge
  - Realistic understanding of options
  - Resources
  - Strengths and limitations

Insight

- Extent of individual's awareness of his or her problem
- Willingness to look at one's role in maintaining symptoms
- Awareness of behavioral consequences and lifestyle changes needed for coping

Screening

The goals of screening and diagnosis differ. Screening is the identification of those persons who possibly have a particular problem. In screening, false positives are acceptable because the goal is to detect all persons at risk and refer them for further analysis and diagnosis. Diagnosis is the process of identifying the correct reason for the symptoms so treatment can begin. In diagnosis we need to be accurate, so false positives are not acceptable.

One of the goals of *Healthy People 2010* (Box 4–2) is to increase early detection and intervention for mental health problems. Screening tools can help practitioners detect people who are at risk for specific mental disorders. An example is the Teen Screen program, developed at Columbia University, for early detection of depression in teens. Screening tools have also been developed for many mental health conditions. Mental health awareness day campaigns provide opportunities for free screening and information for the public. The Joint Commission (2008) advocates screening hospitalized patients for violence risk, psychological trauma history, substance use, and patient strengths. Knowledge of patient strengths is essential for patient-centered care.

Box 4–2. Healthy People 2010: Mental Health Goals

Reduce suicide rate
Reduce homelessness in the mentally ill
Reduce relapse rates
Increase screening
Increase access to treatment
Increase consumer involvement
Cultural competence

Screen for Suicide Risk

Suicide is a public health problem that is the 11th leading cause of death among Americans of all ages and the third leading cause of death among adolescents. Men over the age of 75 have the highest rate of completed suicides and firearms are the most common method used. All individuals in psychiatric care must be screened for suicide risk.
- Suicidal ideation
- Previous attempt, history of abuse or neglect
- History of depression or other mental illness
- Alcohol or drug abuse
- Family history of suicide or violence
- Physical illness
- Feeling alone
- History of or current impulsivity
- Firearms in the home

If a patient acknowledges having thoughts of harming him- or herself or others, assess the level of lethality. Lethality assessments include assessing the intent to die, the severity of the ideation, the availability of means, and the degree of planning. If the patient appears to be acutely suicidal, immediate action is required, including hospitalization, removal of all potentially dangerous objects, and one-on-one observation. No-suicide contracts that require the at-risk patient to commit to not harming him- or herself are often included in inpatient and outpatient care, but the evidence for their efficacy in preventing suicides is weak. Hospital policy determines the protocol for reducing the level of observation as a patient's suicide risk decreases.

Screen for Risk of Violence Toward Others

Violence toward others includes threats (verbal) and acts (physical) directed toward people, animals, or the environment. Escalating youth violence is a major public health concern. The Centers for Disease Control and Prevention (CDC, 2008) reports that among 10–24-year-old males, homicide is the leading cause of death for African Americans, the second leading cause of death for Hispanics and Asian/Pacific Islanders, and the third leading cause of death for Native Americans and Alaskan Natives. Intimate partner violence is a cyclical syndrome involving verbal threats, emotional abuse, and physical and sexual abuse. Although individuals of any age can be abused, children age 4 or younger are the most vulnerable. Child abuse includes physical, sexual, and emotional abuse and neglect. The risk factors for violence and abuse include the following:

- Psychological
  - Severe emotional deprivation or overt rejection in childhood, or parental seduction
  - Exposure to violence in formative years
  - Families with histories of violence, drug abuse, poverty, chronic health problems, or lack of social support
- Physiological
  - Brain damage, mental retardation, learning disabilities that impair capacity to cope with frustration
  - Abuse of alcohol or other disinhibiting substances
- Sociocultural
  - Lack of interpersonal ties
- Behavioral history
  - Childhood cruelty to animals or children
  - Fire-setting or similar dangerous actions
  - Recent violent behavior toward self or others
  - Recent accidents, threats, poor judgment in potentially dangerous situations
- Observable behavior and emotional responses
  - Escalating irritability, sensitivity, or hostility
  - Altered states of consciousness/substance abuse
  - Emotions: severe anger (rage) or fear (panic)
  - Active psychotic symptoms with paranoid ideation

If the problem-based assessments indicate a risk for violence, or if any unusual bruising or injuries are present, further action is required. The nurse has a duty to warn and protect any potential victim of physical violence. The nurse must report any suspected child abuse to Child

Protective Services. Though not mandatory in all states, the nurse should report suspected abuse of elders or vulnerable adults to Adult Protective Services. Finally, the nurse must report gunshot wounds, knife wounds, or other injury that may have resulted from various illegal or unlawful acts.

Screen for Substance Use

Two screening tools commonly used in psychiatric evaluations are the Mini-Mental State Exam (MMSE) and the CAGE questionnaire. The MMSE (Box 4–3) screens for cognitive impairment. It is scored on a scale of 0 to 30, and anyone scoring 24 or less should be further evaluated for medical (dementia, delirium) or substance-related problems. The CAGE questionnaire (Box 4–4) is a 4-item screening tool that detects alcohol (or other substance) problems. A person scoring 1 on the screening should be further assessed for substance problems and a person scoring 2 or more is considered to be positive for a substance disorder.

Box 4–3. MMSE	Box 4–4. CAGE
Orientation (10 pts.) Year, season, date, day, month State, country, town, hospital, floor **Registration** (3 pts.) Name 3 objects **Attention and Calculation** (5 pts.) Serial 7s or "world" spelled backwards **Recall** (3 pts.) Recall the 3 objects **Language** (9 pts.) Name a pencil and watch Repeat "No ifs, ands, or buts" Carry out 3-stage command Read "Close your eyes" Write a sentence Copy overlapping pentagons	• Have you ever felt the need to Cut down on your drinking? • Have you ever felt Annoyed by criticism of drinking? • Have you ever felt Guilty about drinking? • Have you ever taken a drink first thing in the morning (Eye-opener) to steady your nerves or get rid of a hangover?
Normal score: 25–30	Scoring: 2 or more yes is positive for alcohol disorder; 1 yes indicates hazardous drinking.

Box 4–3 adapted from M. Folstein, S. Folstein, & P. McHugh, 1975, "Mini-mental State": A practical method for grading the cognitive state of patients for the clinician, *Journal of Psychiatric Research*, 12, 189–198.

Screen for Dementia

Individuals who score below the normal range on the MMSE (Box 4–3), and upon further assessment do not appear to have substance use problems, should be assessed for dementia. A recent report of the Alzheimer's Foundation (Powers, Ashford, & Peschin, 2008) recommends early detection and treatment of dementia. Unrecognized dementia reduces the autonomy of affected individuals and increases their risks for harm from a variety of causes, including participation in other potentially harmful activities (e.g., driving), noncompliance with prescribed medication regimens, and other difficulties with activities of daily living. Individuals who score within the impaired range of the MMSE and who are also disoriented and confused may have delirium and should be referred for further evaluation.

Screen for Fall Risk

Falls are one of the major sources of injury in older adults. The National Patient Safety Goals, published by The Joint Commission (2009), include reducing the risk of patient harm from falls. Hospitals and long-term-care facilities are required to implement and evaluate fall reduction programs. Many of the psychiatric drugs can cause sedation and therefore increased risk for falls. Other risks for falls include:
- Age over 60: History of falls, smoking, or alcohol or drug abuse
- Mental status: Lethargic, confused or disoriented, inability to understand directions, impaired memory or judgment
- Physical conditions: Acute illness, dehydration, vertigo, unsteady gait, problems affecting weight-bearing joints, weakness, paresis/paralysis, seizure disorder, impaired vision, impaired hearing, slow reaction times, diarrhea, urinary frequency, incontinence, urgency, nocturia, orthostatic hypotension, stroke, musculoskeletal disorders, and Parkinson's disease
- Medications: Diuretics, hypotensives, central nervous system depressants (e.g., benzodiazepines), medications that increase gastrointestinal motility (e.g., laxatives)
- Use of ambulatory devices (indicates problem with walking): Cane, crutches, walker, wheelchair, geri-chair, braces

Screen for Pain

Chronic pain is a risk factor for mood and substance disorders. Historically, pain has been under-recognized and undertreated. The Joint Commission approved new pain assessment and management standards in 1999 that require all healthcare organizations to screen for pain. Unrecognized or undertreated pain may result in psychiatric symptoms such as anxiety, depression, and agitation. If pain is present, a complete assessment follows. The ABCDE approach includes screening, assessment, and treatment.
- **ABCDE**
  - Ask about pain regularly. Assess pain systematically.
  - Believe the client and family in their report of pain and what relieves it.
  - Choose pain control options appropriate for the client, family, and setting.
  - Deliver interventions in a timely, logical, and coordinated fashion.
  - Empower clients and their families. Enable them to control their course to the greatest extent possible.

- **Wong-Baker FACES** scale can be used from age 3 and up.
  - Point to each face using the words to describe the pain intensity.
  - 0 = no hurt (smiling, happy face).
  - 10 = hurts worst (sad, crying face).

Assess Nutritional Status

- Personal information: Age, activity level, cultural background, socioeconomic status, personal preferences, use of alcohol or illegal drugs, supplements, prescriptions
- Body mass index (BMI): Can be calculated from height and weight
- Body weight within norms for gender/age/height
- Body weight 15% or more below expected weight should receive further work-up
- 24-hour food history/diary
- Fluid intake: Food diary: 3–7 days. Calculate nutritional intake and compare it with USDA daily reference values to determine whether dietary habits are adequate.
- Knowledge of nutrition

Assess Physical Status

Vital Signs and Labs. See Table 4–1 for a description of normal vital sign levels and common laboratory values. Specific lab tests may be ordered to rule out alcohol or drug abuse or other medical disorders prior to making a psychiatric diagnosis.

Table 4–1. Normal Values for Vital Signs and Labs

Normal Vital Signs	Normal Lab Values (Fasting)

• Temperature
  - Oral: 37°C/98.6°F
• Pulse rate
  - Infant: 120–160 bpm
  - Child: 75–100 bpm
  - Adolescent: 60–90 bpm
  - Adult: 60–100 bpm
• Blood pressure
  - 1 yr: 95/65
  - 10 yrs: 110/65
  - Adolescent: 120/75
  - Adult: 120/80
  - Elder: 140/90
  - Hypertension (adult): 140–159/90–99
• Respiratory rate (breaths/min)
  - 6 mos: 30–50
  - 2 yrs: 25–32
  - Child: 20–30
  - Adolescent: 16–19
  - Adult: 12–20
	• Complete blood cell count with differential
	  - WBC: 3,300–9,600 µL
	  - Agranulocytosis: WBC is <2,000 X µL
	• Thyroid function tests
	  - TSH: 0.43–4.6 µIU/mL
	• Liver function
	  - ALT (SGOT): 0–40 IU/L
	  - AST (SGPT): 0–40 IU/L
	  - Bilirubin: 0.1–1.2 mg/dL
	• Kidney function
	  - Creatinine clearance: 0.5–1.5 mg/dL
	  - BUN (elevated in renal disease): 5–26 mg/dL
	• Glucose
	  - 70–115 mg/dL
	
	Examples of other labs that may be ordered include medication levels, drug toxicology screens, and serum albumin.

General Functioning and Review of Systems

The *general survey* involves observing the patient for age-appropriate appearance, behaviors, and developmental milestones. We also observe the patient's interactions with family members, or others if present. Physical observation of the patient is part of the MSE.

- *Infants:* Observe parent–infant interactions, feeding, nutritional state, and cry
- *Early childhood:* Observe mood, nutritional state, speech, cry, facial expression, apparent emotional and chronologic age, skills, parent–child interactions, separation, tolerance, affection, and discipline
- *Late childhood:* Observe orientation to time and place, factual knowledge, language and number skills, motor skills used in writing, tying laces, buttoning, and drawing
- *Adult:* Observe general state of health, height, build, sexual development, posture, motor activity, gait, dress, grooming, personal hygiene, odors, affect, reactions, speech, level of consciousness, and mental status

The *review of the systems* documents the presence or absence of common symptoms related to each major body system. In the review of symptoms, we simply ask about any bothersome symptoms, generally proceeding from head to toe: "How is your/your child's...?" We also inquire about functional health patterns as part of the psychiatric and medical history (see Table 4–2).

Table 4-2. System Review

Physical Systems	Functional Health Patterns
Neurological	Health perception/health management
Endocrine	Nutritional-metabolic
Respiratory	Elimination
Cardiovascular	Activity-exercise
Gastrointestinal	Cognitive-perceptual
Genitourinary	Sleep-rest
Musculoskeletal	Self-perception/self-concept
Integumentary	Sexuality-reproductive
Hematologic	Coping-stress-tolerance
	Value-belief

Identifying functional strengths as well as weaknesses assists in care planning. The DSM-IV-TR's *Global Assessment of Functioning Scale* (GAF) provides a scale for estimating overall psychosocial functioning and monitoring change. The scale ranges from 1–10 ("persistent danger of severely hurting self or others") to 91–100 ("superior functioning in a wide range of activities, life's problems never seem to get out of hand, is sought out by others because of his or her many positive qualities"). Individuals with a GAF of 30 or less are unable to care for themselves ("behavior is considerably influenced by delusions or hallucinations...or inability to function in almost all areas"). See Table 4–6 for more information on coding the GAF.

A physical examination is completed within 24 hours of admission to the psychiatric hospital or care facility. It generally proceeds from head to toe, using techniques of auscultation (listening), inspection (observation), palpation (touch), and percussion (tapping). The MSE is a component of the neurological exam. The neurological exam also includes assessment of reflexes, muscle strength, coordination, balance, and sensation. The cranial nerves (Box 4–5) are examined by observing sense of smell, eye movements, strength of the temporal and masseter muscles, corneal reflexes, facial movements, gag reflex, and strength of the trapezia and sternomastoidal muscles. While conducting a review of systems, or physical exam of the psychiatric patient, it is important to be aware of potential associated symptoms, or medication side effects that may present. Examples of abnormal physical findings are listed in Table 4–5. These symptoms, if present, should be evaluated in more detail to determine whether they are contributing to psychiatric symptoms, whether they are side effects from medication, or whether they are due to some other cause. Regardless of the cause, most of the symptoms can be treated, so it is important to refer patients for a more complete physical examination if any abnormal physical symptoms are found.

Box 4–5. Cranial Nerves

Olfactory, optic, occulomotor, trochlear, trigeminal, abducens, facial, vestibulochoclear, glosopharyngeal, vagus, accessory, hypoglossal. (For those interested, there are many mneumonics online for memorizing the cranial nerves.)

DIAGNOSIS

The diagnosis is based upon an analysis and synthesis of the collected data and the recognition of functional patterns and trends. An accurate diagnosis guides the direction of treatment and evaluation of care outcomes.

Classification Systems

Several diagnostic classification systems exist for the mental disorders. The North American Nursing Diagnosis Association (NANDA) classification system was developed by nurses to identify problems treatable by nurses. The *Diagnostic and Statistical Manual of Mental Disorders* (DSM-IV-TR; American Psychiatric Association, 2000) used by most psychiatric providers is fully compatible with the World Health Organization's *International Classification for Diseases* control codes (ICD) required by Medicare and Medicaid.

NANDA: Nursing diagnoses, unlike DSM-IV-TR diagnoses, identify the patient's response, not the medical diagnosis. They are based upon the conceptualization of the human response to actual or potential health problems from the unique nursing perspective. A partial list of NANDA-approved diagnoses that might apply to patients with mental disorders includes:

- Anxiety
- Coping (ineffective, readiness for enhanced, compromised family, defensive)
- Denial, ineffective
- Family processes (dysfunctional, interrupted, readiness for enhanced)
- Fatigue
- Fear
- Grieving (anticipatory, dysfunctional)
- Health maintenance, ineffective
- Health-seeking behavior
- Hopelessness
- Identity, disturbed personal
- Loneliness, risk for
- Memory, impaired
- Pain (acute, chronic)
- Parenting (readiness for enhanced, impaired, risk for impaired)
- Posttrauma syndrome or risk
- Rape-trauma syndrome
- Relocation stress syndrome or risk
- Role performance, ineffective
- Self-care deficit (bathing, dressing, feeding, etc.)
- Self-esteem (chronic low, situational low, risk for low)
- Self-mutilation or risk for
- Sensory perception, disturbed
- Sexual dysfunction
- Sexuality pattern, disturbed
- Sleep pattern, disturbed
- Social interaction, impaired
- Social isolation
- Sorrow, chronic
- Spiritual distress (risk, readiness)
- Suicide risk
- Thought process disturbed
- Violence (risk for other- or self-directed)
- Wandering

DSM-IV-TR provides a "multi-axial" classification system for psychiatric problems:
- *Axis I:* Clinical disorders
  - The focus of clinical attention
- *Axis II:* Personality disorders and mental retardation
  - More long-standing and inflexible mental conditions, not usually the focus of clinical attention, especially in inpatient settings
- *Axis III:* General medical conditions
  - Medical conditions that might have some impact upon the Axis I disorder (e.g., pain conditions, Parkinson's, endocrine disorders)
- *Axis IV:* Psychosocial and environmental problems
  - Significant stressors that may be contributing to the development or exacerbation of the Axis I disorder
- *Axis V:* Global assessment of functioning (GAF)
  - Score of 0–100 indicates general level of functioning

Axis I: Clinical Disorders

Table 4–3 contains a list of mental disorders, along with criteria that are used for determining DSM-IV-TR diagnoses. Advanced practice psychiatric nurses are qualified to make psychiatric diagnoses. In practice, the psychiatric DSM-IV-TR diagnoses are important for determining proper medication regimens; however, they are not as important for determining the non-pharmacological plan of care. The focus of non-pharmacological care, importantly nursing care, is based upon the conceptualization of the human response to actual or potential health problems.

Table 4-3. Symptomatology and Diagnostic Criteria of Axis I Disorder

DSM-IV-TR Diagnosis	Diagnostic Criteria

Thought Disorders
• Schizophrenia
• Schizoaffective disorder
• Brief psychotic disorder
• Schizophreniform disorder
• Shared psychotic disorder
• Delusional disorder
• Psychotic disorder
• Induced psychotic disorder
	Schizophrenia
	• Two or more of the following symptoms have been present for a significant portion of time during a 1-month period
	  - Delusions
	  - Hallucinations
	  - Disorganized speech
	  - Disorganized behavior
	  - Negative symptoms
	• Continuous social/occupational dysfunction for at least 6 months
	• Types: paranoid, disorganized, catatonic, or undifferentiated

Mood Disorders
• Major depression
• Dysthymia
• Bipolar I
• Bipolar II
• Cyclothymia
	Major Depression
	• Five or more symptoms that have been present for 2 weeks or more and represent a change from previous functioning
	• At least one of the symptoms is depressed mood or loss of pleasure
	  - Weight loss
	  - Insomnia or hypersomnia
	  - Psychomotor agitation or retardation
	  - Fatigue or loss of energy
	  - Feelings of worthlessness or excessive guilt
	  - Diminished ability to think or concentrate
	  - Recurrent thoughts of death
	
	Bipolar I (Manic Episode)
	• Presence of current or previous manic episode
	• A distinct period of abnormally and persistently elevated, expansive, or irritable mood, lasting at least 1 week, characterized by 3 or more of the following:
	  - Inflated self-esteem
	  - Decreased need for sleep
	  - More talkative than usual
	  - Flight of ideas
	  - Distractibility
	  - Increase in goal-directed activity
	  - Excessive involvement in pleasurable activities

Continued

Table 4–3. Symptomatology and Diagnostic Criteria of Axis I Disorder (cont.)

Anxiety Disorders	**Panic Disorder**

• Panic disorder
• Generalized anxiety disorder (GAD)
• Phobia
• Obsessive compulsive disorder (OCD)
• Posttraumatic stress disorder (PTSD)
• Separation anxiety disorder (see Disorders of Childhood)
	• Recurrent, unexpected panic attacks
	• At least one of the attacks has been followed by 1 month of:
	  - Persistent concern about having additional attacks
	  - Worry about implications (i.e., losing control, having a heart attack)

GAD
- Excessive anxiety and worry (occurring more days than not for at least 6 months, about a number of events or activities)
- The anxiety and worry are associated with 3 or more of the following 6 symptoms:
  - Restlessness
  - Being easily fatigued
  - Difficulty concentrating
  - Irritability
  - Muscle tension
  - Sleep disturbance

Phobia: Specific, Social, or Agoraphobia
- Marked or persistent fear that is excessive or unreasonable, cued by the presence or anticipation of a specific object or situation
- Exposure to the phobic stimulus almost invariably provokes an immediate anxiety response, which may take the form of a panic attack
- The person recognizes that the fear is excessive
- The phobic stimulus is avoided

OCD
- Either obsessions or compulsions that cause marked distress, are time-consuming, and interfere with functioning
  - Obsessions: recurrent and persistent thoughts, impulses, or images that are intrusive and inappropriate
  - Compulsions: repetitive behaviors that the person feels driven to perform; aimed at anxiety reduction

PTSD
- Person has been exposed to a traumatic event
- The traumatic event is persistently re-experienced
- Persistent avoidance of stimuli associated with the trauma and numbing of general responsiveness
- Persistent symptoms of increased arousal
- Duration is >1 month

Continued

Table 4-3. Symptomatology and Diagnostic Criteria of Axis I Disorder (cont.)

Substance Disorders	Abuse

• Alcohol
• Cocaine
• Inhalants
• Opioids
• Amphetamines, related substances
• Phencyclidines, related substances
• Sedatives, hypnotics, anxiolytics
• Caffeine
• Hallucinogens
• Nicotine
• Some over-the-counter (OTC) combinations
	• Administration of any drug in a culturally disapproved manner that causes adverse consequences
	• Recurrent use causing
	  - Failure in role responsibilities
	  - Physically hazardous situations
	  - Legal problems
	• Continued use despite social and interpersonal problems
	
	Dependence
	• Physical dependence
	  - A physiologic state of neuro-adaptation produced by repeated administration of a drug, necessitating continued administration to prevent withdrawal syndrome
	  - Tolerance: need for increasing amounts for desired effect
	• Psychological dependence
	  - Repeats use to produce pleasure or avoid discomfort
	  - Cravings for drug
	• Substance is often taken in larger amounts or over a longer period than intended
	• Time is spent in activities necessary to obtain the substance
	• Social, occupational, recreational activities given up because of use
	• Unsuccessful efforts to cut down use
	
	Intoxication
	• Reversible substance-specific syndrome caused by substance ingestion
	• Maladaptive behavior due to substances
	• Symptoms not due to medical conditions or other mental disorder
	
	Withdrawal
	• Substance-specific syndrome caused by cessation of prolonged and heavy use
	• Substance-specific syndrome causing impairment in social, occupational, and other areas of functioning
	• Symptoms not due to medical condition or accounted for by other mental disorder
	• Withdrawal symptoms are generally the opposite of intoxication symptoms

Continued

Table 4–3. Symptomatology and Diagnostic Criteria of Axis I Disorder (cont.)

Disorders Beginning in Childhood

Anxiety	**Separation Anxiety Disorder** • Developmentally inappropriate and excessive anxiety concerning separation from home or attachment figures • Persistent worry, reluctance to go to school, etc. • Repeated nightmares • Repeated somatic symptoms • Onset prior to age 18
Pervasive Developmental Disorders (Autism Spectrum Disorders) • Autistic disorder • Asperger syndrome • Rett syndrome • Childhood disintegrative disorder • Pervasive developmental disorder	**Autism** • Qualitative impairment in social interaction • Qualitative impairments in communication • Restricted, repetitive, and stereotyped patterns of behavior, interests, and activities • Delays or abnormal functioning in at least one of the following, with onset prior to age 3: - Social interaction - Language - Symbolic or imaginative play
ADHD (Attention-Deficit Hyperactivity Disorder)	**ADHD** • Six or more symptoms of inattention have persisted for at least 6 months to a degree that is maladaptive and inconsistent with developmental level • Six or more symptoms of hyperactivity-impulsivity have persisted for at least 6 months to a degree that is maladaptive and inconsistent with developmental level • Symptoms that caused impairment were present before age 7
Disorders of Conduct	**Oppositional Defiant Disorder** • A pattern of negativistic, hostile, and defiant behavior - Loses temper, argues, annoys, blames, easily annoyed **Conduct Disorder** • A repetitive and persistent pattern of behavior in which the basic rights of others, or societal norms or rules, are violated - Aggression toward people or animals - Destruction of property - Deceitfulness or theft - Serious violations of rules

Continued

Table 4-3. Symptomatology and Diagnostic Criteria of Axis I Disorder (cont.)

Eating Disorders	**Bulimia**
	• Recurrent episodes of binge eating
	  - Eating greater amounts than most people
	  - Sense of lack of control
	• Recurrent, inappropriate compensatory behavior
	• Compensatory behaviors at least 2x/wk for 3 months
	• Purging type or nonpurging type

	Anorexia • Refusal to maintain body weight at or above 85% of expected • Intense fear of gaining weight • Disturbance in self-perception • Amenorrhea for at least 2 consecutive cycles • Restricting or binge/purge types
Disorders Associated With Aging	

Cognitive Disorders	**Dementia**
	• Onset (usually gradual) of multiple cognitive deficits, including memory loss and at least one of the following:
	  - Aphasia
	  - Apraxia
	  - Agnosia
	  - Disturbed executive functioning
	• Impairment in social or occupational functioning

	Delirium • A disturbance in consciousness that is accompanied by a change in cognition that cannot be better accounted for by a preexisting or evolving dementia • Acute confusion • Disturbance develops over a short period of time (usually hours to days) and tends to fluctuate during the course of the day • May demonstrate psychomotor agitation or depression

Culturally Specific Disorders

Cultural factors affect the expression and prevalence of mental disorders, as well as the interpretation of assessment data and treatment options. Several culturally specific formulations are listed within the DSM-IV-TR:

- *Acculturation problem:* The focus of clinical attention is a problem involving adjustment to a different culture
- *Culture-bound syndromes:* Mental disorders particular to certain cultures

- Examples: Amok (Malaysia), Brain Fag (West Africa), Ataque de nervios (Latin America), and Evil Eye (Mediterranean cultures)

Axis II: Personality Disorders

Personality is the enduring pattern of inner experience and behavior that is established in the late teens or early adulthood. Personality disorders (see Table 4–4) are diagnosed when people experience clinically significant distress or impairment related to longstanding inflexible and pervasive patterns. Problematic behaviors are manifested in two or more of the following:

- Cognition (ways of perceiving and interpreting self, other people, and events)
- Affectivity (the range, intensity, lability, and appropriateness of emotional response)
- Interpersonal functioning
- Impulse control

Table 4–4. Characteristics of Axis II Personality Disorders

Cluster	Type
Cluster A: Odd & Eccentric	**Paranoid:** Suspicious, mistrustful, appears defensive or resistant to control, very skeptical of most things, copes by projection, attributes shortcomings to others to justify actions **Schizoid:** Asocial pattern: aloof, introverted, seclusive, uninterested in social activities, apathetic, unengaged; thought to be schizophrenic prodrome; copes by intellectualizing **Schizotypal:** Odd, bizarre, strange, magical, eccentric, socially anxious, secretive and private, copes by undoing, easily overwhelmed by stimulation; many bizarre acts/thoughts reflect a retraction of previous acts/thoughts
Cluster B: Dramatic & Emotional	**Antisocial:** The psychopath; delinquent, criminal; lack of superego; impulsive; thrill-seeking, irresponsible; get pleasure from swindling others; copes by acting out. **Borderline:** Unstable, intense affect, impulsivity with self-damaging acts, identity disturbance, chaotic relationships, manipulativeness, abandonment concerns, demanding, unpredictable, "black or white," "all or nothing"; copes by regression, projection, and denial **Histrionic:** Gregarious, seductive, dramatic, tendency to sexualize all relationships, extreme extraversion, attention-seeking, superficial, difficulty in maintaining deep relationships; copes by creating facades **Narcissistic:** Egotistical, preoccupied with power and prestige, sense of superiority, arrogant, entitled; copes by rationalizing, repressing, and using fantasy

Continued

Table 4-4. Characteristics of Axis II Personality Disorders (cont.)

Cluster C:	**Avoidant:** Withdrawn pattern, sensitive to rejection/humiliation, slow and constrained speech, shy and uncomfortable with others, sees self as inferior; copes by using fantasy and daydreams
Anxious & Fearful	**Dependent:** Submissive pattern, need for social approval, clingy, feels inadequate, wants others to manage life, relates to others in an immature and child-like way, naïve; copes by using introjection—internalizing beliefs of others
	Obsessive Compulsive: Conforming, meticulous, rigid, disciplined, concerned with order and conformity, stubborn, usually copes by using reaction-formation (doing the opposite of their feelings), isolation, and undoing

Axis III: General Medical Conditions

Axis III lists any physical disorder or general medical condition that is present in addition to the mental disorder. The physical condition may be causative, the result of a mental disorder, or unrelated. Table 4–5 shows examples of physical conditions that may be present in individuals who have mental disorders.

Table 4-5. Examples of Abnormal Physical Findings Related to Mental Disorders or Treatments

Functional System	Symptoms	Possible Mechanism
Head	Progressively severe headache: Eyes (and vision)	Hypertensive crisis due to tyramine interaction with monoamine oxidase inhibitors (MAOIs)
Eyes and Vision	Nystagmus	Substance intoxication, brain lesions
	Oculogyric crisis	Neuroleptic induced dystonia
Ears and Hearing	Diminished hearing	Age-related diminished hearing may be misinterpreted as cognitive impairment in older adults
Throat and Neck	High fever and sore throat	Agranulocytosis (greatest risk with Clozapine)
	Thyroid enlargement (goiter)	Hypothyroidism

Continued

Table 4–5. Examples of Abnormal Physical Findings Related to Mental Disorders or Treatments (cont.)

Respiratory system	Anxiety	Hyperventilation, asthma, shortness of breath
Integumentary System	Rash	Possible allergic reaction Risk for Stevens-Johnson syndrome (toxic epidermal necrolysis) if on lamotrigine.
Neurological System	Tremors	Lithium: Fine motor Parkinson's: Slow resting Anticonvulsants: Fine motor
	Gait and balance disturbances	Encephalopathy, intoxication, cerebellar injuries
	Disorientation, confusion	Delirium, anticholinergic toxicity
	Weakness, numbness	Cerebrovascular events
	Anxiety	Drug intoxication or withdrawal, stimulants, seizures
Cardiovascular	ECG changes	Tricyclics, anticholinergics, some antipsychotics (e.g., Geodon)
	Orthostatic hypotension	Tricyclics, antipsychotics, antihypertensives
	Tachycardia	Anxiety, stimulants, anorexia
	Hypertension	Antipsychotics (metabolic syndrome) MAOI-induced hypertensive crisis
	Bradycardia	Beta-blockers, anorexia, Parkinson's
	Anxiety	Anemia, angina, congestive heart failure, mitral valve prolapse, tachycardia
Gastrointestinal (GI) system	GI distress, nausea	Lithium: Recommend taking with food SSRIs: Especially early in treatment

Continued

**Table 4–5. Examples of Abnormal Physical Findings Related
to Mental Disorders or Treatments (cont.)**

Endocrine System	Abnormal glucose metabolism	Antipsychotics (metabolic syndrome)
	Hyperprolactinemia	Can be a side effect of antipsychotic dopaminergic blockade
	Depression	Hypothyroidism, chronically elevated cortisol (prolonged stress response)
	Anxiety	Hyperthyroidism, hypoglycemia, premenstrual syndrome
Genitourinary System	Polyuria, polydipsia	Lithium adverse affect. Renal disease or drugs that reduce renal clearance (e.g., NSAIDs) may increase serum concentration of drugs that are excreted by the kidneys (e.g., lithium)
	Unusual pattern of bruises or trauma	Rule out sexual or physical abuse
	Sexual dysfunction	May be side effect from antihypertensives, antidepressants, antihistamines, or antispasmodics
	Delirium	Kidney failure
Musculoskeletal System	Body asymmetry	Dystonias (muscle spasms as a result of Parkinsonism side effects), CVAs, lesions
	Abnormal movements: dyskinesias, dystonia, bradykinesia, akathesia	Parkinson's and Parkinsonism related to antipsychotic extrapyramidal side effects
	Gait disturbances	Cerebellar dysfunction such as seen with alcoholic encephalopathy (Wernicke's), substance use disorders
	Swallowing problems	Parkinson's disease, advanced dementia, antipsychotic-induced dystonias

Axis IV: Psychosocial and Environmental Problems

Psychosocial and environmental problems judged to be contributing to the clinical disorder are coded on Axis IV. Stress may arise from any of the following categories with examples:
- Primary support group: Death, health problems, abuse, dysfunction
- Social environment: Death of friend, living alone, discrimination
- Education: Illiteracy, academic problems, inadequate school environment, discord with teachers or fellow students
- Occupation: Unemployment, job dissatisfaction, job change, discord with boss or coworkers
- Housing: Homelessness, inadequate housing, unsafe neighborhood
- Economic: Extreme poverty, inadequate finances, insufficient welfare support
- Access to health care: Inadequate or unavailable care, inadequate transportation or health insurance
- Other: Exposure to disasters, war, or discord with nonfamily caregivers

Axis V: Global Assessment of Functioning

The Global Assessment of Functioning (GAF) is useful for documenting baseline functioning and tracking progress with treatment. The GAF measurement is generally coded for the period of time surrounding the evaluation, although an estimate is sometimes made about previous periods of time for comparison (e.g., the last year). The GAF is determined by the scale range (see Table 4–6) that matches the individual's symptom severity OR the level of functioning (e.g., social, occupational, school), whichever is worse.

Table 4–6. Coding Global Assessment of Functioning by Symptom Severity and Level of Functioning

Code	Symptom Severity	Level of Functioning
91-100	No symptoms	Superior functioning
81-90	Absent or minimal symptoms	Good functioning
71-80	Transient and expectable reactions to psychosocial stressors	No more than slight functional impairment in social, occupation, or school
61-70	Mild symptoms	Generally functioning pretty well, with some difficulties
51-60	Moderate symptoms	Moderate difficulty in functioning
41-50	Serious symptoms (e.g., suicidal ideation)	Serious impairment in functioning
31-40	Some impairment in reality testing or communication	Major problems in functioning

Continued

Table 4–6. Coding Global Assessment of Functioning by Symptom Severity and Level of Functioning (cont.)

21-30	Behavior is influenced by delusions or hallucinations or serious impairment in communication	Inability to function in almost all areas
11-20	Some danger of hurting self or others or gross impairment in communication	Major problems in functioning; occasionally fails to maintain hygiene
0-10	Persistent danger of severely hurting self or others	Inability to maintain minimal personal hygiene or serious suicidal act with clear expectations of death

OUTCOME IDENTIFICATION

In 2003, the New Freedom Commission on Mental Health called for a fundamental transformation of the mental health delivery system, calling for a shift to self-management and recovery from mental illness. Recovery does not necessarily mean "cure," but it does mean the ability to live a fulfilling and productive life despite a disability. Self-determination is an important component of recovery. In the context of recovery-based care, the nurse involves patients and their families in healthcare decision-making to set mutually agreeable goals and develop a realistic plan of action.

Categories of outcome indicators include clinical, functional, satisfaction, and financial. Separate outcomes are identified for each identified problem. Good outcomes are:
- Measurable: Standardized outcome measures are best
- Specific: Quality, quantity, severity, and frequency
- Time-limited: Determine short- and long-term goals
- Realistic within the time specified with a consideration of benefits and costs
- Evidence-based

Use Standardized Measures When Possible

Standardized psychometric rating scales can help add more specificity to findings of symptoms and can be used to evaluate responses to treatment. A variety of standardized assessment scales are in the public domain.

PLANNING

The first step in planning care is to identify the priorities for treatment. Highest priority is given to conditions that, if untreated, could result in harm. These would include those that involve basic survival needs or safety needs related to SI or HI, or threat of harm from others (e.g., domestic violence, child abuse). Intermediate priority is given to nonemergent, non–life-threatening, but distressing, painful, or dysfunctional symptoms (e.g., hallucinations, agitation). Lower priority is given to issues that are not specifically related to the illness or prognosis (e.g., occupational, social stressors). Maslow's Hierarchy of Needs (Figure 4–1) can be used to conceptualize the priorities for care planning.

Figure 4–1. Maslow's Hierarchy of Needs

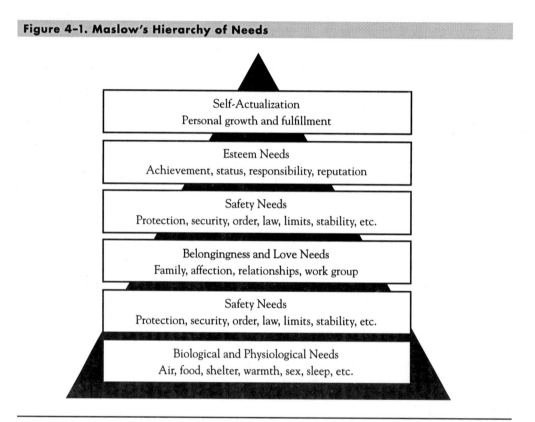

Adapted from *Motivation and personality* (rev. ed.) by A. Maslow, 1970, New York: Harper & Row.

The treatment plan specifies, by priority, the diagnoses, short-term and long-term goals/ expected outcomes, and the interventions, including the what, when, where, how, and who. When available, predeveloped, current, evidence-based practice guidelines, clinical pathways, or clinical algorithms can be used. When new or unusual care needs arise, the nurse is advised to utilize current research (Chapter 11) to identify evidence-based approaches.

Case Management. Case management includes the development of a plan of care to meet identified needs, ensuring access to care, and implementing a method of monitoring care. Case managers understand and can work between and within systems, connecting services and acting as an important safety net in the event of a service gap. Case managers can be helpful in determining the best location for care, based upon individual needs. Formalized case management falls within the scope of the advanced practice psychiatric–mental health nurse (ANA, 2007).

IMPLEMENTATION

Interventions at the Biological or Physiological Level

At the level of biological and physiological needs, interventions support physiological functioning. Biological treatments may include interventions involving self-care activities, exercise or activities, sleep, nutrition and hydration, pain management, relaxation training, and medication management.

Interventions at the Level of Safety

Provide Safety. Once the patient is stable, interventions turn to safety. Nurses structure the milieu to provide safety as well as opportunities for group activities and positive social interactions. When a patient is threatening the safety of the milieu, nursing interventions focus on reducing the likelihood of harm.
- Reduce stimulation in the milieu
- Remove lethal material
- Separate from other patients
- Contract for safety
- Constant one-on-one monitoring
- Maintain safety: observe for escalation
- Remain calm: defuse with least restrictive means

Use De-escalating Communication Strategies.
- Speak in a calm, low voice
- Respect need for personal space
- Avoid intense eye contact
- Acknowledge the patient's feelings and reassure that staff are there to help
- Communicate expected behavior
- Communicate consequences of unacceptable behavior
- Give opportunity for time out

Use Seclusion or Restraints Only if Necessary. In high-risk, potentially violent, or life-threatening situations where preventive and de-escalating strategies have failed, seclusion or restraints might be required.
- Requires a team response with a designated team leader
- Notify security if necessary
- Remove all other patients from the area
- The leader expresses concern for the patient's safety and behavior

- At given signal, team secures the patient's limbs
- Patient is escorted to appropriate room and informed of the intervention
- If necessary, restraints or medications are administered

The Centers for Medicare and Medicaid Services (CMS) have established required guidelines for the use of seclusion or restraints to reduce the risk of harming the patients. Anyone restrained must be evaluated by a physician or licensed independent practitioner within 1 hour. The patient must be monitored continuously and the procedure must be terminated as soon as the patient meets the criteria for release. The nurse must document the behaviors, the attempts to use less restrictive interventions, the nursing care provided, the patient's response to the treatments, and the rationale for terminating the intervention.

Interventions at the Level of Psychosocial Needs

At this level, interventions support psychosocial functioning and facilitate lifestyle changes. This is really the working phase of a therapeutic relationship. Interventions can include behavioral therapy, cognitive therapy, communication enhancement, coping assistance, patient education, and psychological comfort promotion. The family may be included in some of the counseling and education interventions. Specific psychosocial interventions are reviewed in Chapters 8 and 9.

Interventions at the Levels of Esteem Needs and Self-Actualization

A recovery-based mental health system addresses self-esteem and self-actualization needs by treating patients with dignity and respect, including them as essential partners in the healthcare team, and empowering them to regain control over their lives and return to previous higher levels of functioning. Self-determination includes giving individuals the freedom to choose where and with whom one lives as well as how one organizes all important aspects of one's life with freely chosen assistance as needed. Individuals must be given the authority, support, and responsibility to make choices about how healthcare dollars are spent on their behalf.

EVALUATION OF OUTCOMES

Evaluation begins with the formation of measurable outcome goals.

Evaluation is systematic, ongoing, and criterion-based. Any of the following types of information may be used to evaluate individual response to treatment:
- Physical exam findings: Examples include weight changes, strength, endurance, and blood pressure
- Mental status changes: Examples include thought process and content
- Laboratory test results: Examples include drug levels, blood glucose levels

- Scores on rating scales: Examples of scales that are used to evaluate the response to nursing care or medications include:
  - *Abnormal Involuntary Movement Scale* (AIMS; Guy, 1976). This scale is useful for quantifying the presence of extrapyramidal side effects in individuals who are taking antipsychotics. The presence and severity of each potential abnormal movement is rated from none to severe:
    - sitting, standing, walking
    - tongue, mouth
    - rapid finger-thumb tapping
    - passive flexion and extension of the arms
  - *The Clinical Institute Withdrawal Assessment for Alcohol Withdrawal* (CIWA-A; Shaw, Kolesar, Sellers, Kaplan, & Sandor, 1981) is an instrument that helps in the assessment of alcohol withdrawal and serves as a guide in the treatment of the condition. During detoxification from alcohol, CIWA-A scores are determined every 30 minutes until the scores are reduced to <10 for 3 consecutive assessments or for 4 hours.
  - *The Brief Psychiatric Rating Scale* (BPRS; Overall, 1988) is an 18-item scale measuring positive symptoms, affective symptoms, and general psychopathology. It can be rated on observation of the patient and can be used to monitor outcomes of treatment.

Evaluation is the last step of the nursing process as it is the last step of the evidence-based care process. That is not to say that evaluation is the end of either process. Providing evidence-based nursing care is circular. As we evaluate outcomes, we revise our care plans as necessary until the goals for treatment are met. More details of outcome evaluation are available in Chapter 11.

REFERENCES

American Nurses Association and American Psychiatric Nurses Association. (2007). *Psychiatric–mental health nursing: Scope and standards of practice.* Silver Spring, MD: American Nurses Association.

American Psychiatric Association. (2000). *Diagnostic and statistical manual of mental disorders* (4th ed., text rev.). Washington, DC: Author.

Centers for Disease Control and Prevention. (2006–2008). *Injury center: Facts at a glance.* Retrieved November 28, 2008, from http://www.cdc.gov/ncipc/dvp/CMP/default.htm

Folstein, M., Folstein, S., & McHugh, P. (1975). "Mini-mental State": A practical method for grading the cognitive state of patients for the clinician. *Journal of Psychiatric Research, 12,* 189–198.

Guy, W. (1976). ECDEU: *Assessment manual for psychopharmacology* (DHEW Publication No. 76-338). Washington, DC: Department of Health, Education, and Welfare, Psychopharmacology Research Branch.

The Joint Commission. (2008). *Specifications manual for national hospital inpatient quality measures: Hospital-based inpatient psychiatric services core measurement set.* Verson 2.0. Oakbrook Terrace, IL: Author.

The Joint Commission. (2009). *National patient safety goals.* Retrieved January 18, 2009, from http://www.jointcommission.org/PatientSafety/NationalPatientSafetyGoals/

Maslow, A. (1970). *Motivation and personality* (rev. ed.). New York: Harper & Row.

NANDA International. (2008). *Nursing diagnoses. Definitions and classification 2009–2011.* Indianapolis: Wiley-Blackwell.

New Freedom Commission on Mental Health (2003). *Achieving the promise: Transforming mental health care in America.* Final report, DHHS Pub. No. SMA-03-3832. Rockville, MD: U.S. Department of Health and Human Services.

Overall, J. (1988). The Brief Psychiatric Rating Scale (BPRS): Recent developments in ascertainment and scaling. *Psychopharmacology Bulletin, 24,* 97–99.

Powers, R. E., Ashford, J. W., & Peschin, S. (2008). *Memory matters. Screening approaches to increase early detection and treatment of Alzheimer's disease and related dementias, and recommendations for national policy.* New York: Alzheimer's Foundation of America.

Shaw, J., Kolesar, G., Sellers, E., Kaplan, H., & Sandor, P. (1981). Development of optimal treatment tactics for alcohol withdrawal, I: Assessment and effectiveness of supportive care. *Journal of Clinical Psychopharmacology, 8,* 382–389.

U.S. Department of Health and Human Services, Office of Disease Prevention and Health Promotion (n.d.). *Healthy People 2010.* Retrieved November 20, 2008, from http://www.healthypeople.gov

Provision of Care

Elizabeth Arnold, PhD, RN, PMHCNS-BC

Chapter 5 sets forth the key professional, legal, ethical, and regulatory standards needed to ensure the quality and provision of safe, effective nursing care. The chapter reviews reimbursement structures currently in place to provide cost-effective, quality care, and identifies the major accrediting bodies relevant to the provision of care in psychiatric–mental health nursing.

FACTORS AFFECTING SCOPE OF PRACTICE

Several factors affect the actual scope of practice for psychiatric–mental health nurses, including licensure and allowable practices within particular clinical settings. The American Nurses Association's *Social Policy Statement* (2003) and Institute of Medicine (2001) recommendations for patient-centered care broaden the nurse's understanding of published professional standards of psychiatric nursing practice and professional performance.

State Licensure

Although the overarching scope of practice for psychiatric–mental health nurses is established by the profession and is published through the professional association for nurses, the American

Nurses Association (ANA), specific guidelines and licensure requirements are state regulated through each state's Board of Nursing. "Boards of Nursing are state governmental agencies that are responsible for the regulation of nursing practice in each respective state. Boards of Nursing are authorized to enforce the Nurse Practice Act, develop administrative rules/regulations and other responsibilities per the Nurse Practice Act" (National Council of State Boards of Nursing, 2008). Each state has its own requirements, rules, and regulations for nursing practice. Scope of practice regulations differ for basic and advanced practice nurses in most states. Nurses are responsible for practicing in accordance with state laws.

Multistate Licensure

Registered nurses legally residing in a nurse licensure compact state are eligible for multistate professional licenses. A mutual recognition model of nurse licensure, multistate licensing is the result of legislative action to allow professional nurses to practice across state lines without having to secure a separate license in each state. This model allows a nurse to have one license (in his or her state of residency) and to practice in other compact states (both physically and electronically) without needing to secure an additional RN license. The nurse is subject to each state's practice laws and discipline. Under mutual recognition, a nurse may practice across state lines unless otherwise restricted. The state of residence, not the state of practice, determines the licensure-granting state. Over the past few years, more than half the nation's states have enacted the RN and LPN/VN nurse licensure compact.

Clinical Practice Settings

Psychiatric–mental health nurses may practice in organized clinical settings, where they work as salaried or fee-for-service employees. Advanced practice nurses may also be self-employed and practice autonomously. Common practice settings include:
- Crisis intervention and psychiatric emergency care services
- Acute intensive care units within a psychiatric or general hospital
- Intermediate and long-term-care facilities
- Partial hospitalization
- Residential facilities for chronically ill patients
- Intensive outpatient treatment
- Community mental health centers
- Detoxification and substance abuse treatment centers
- Shelters, group homes
- Assertive Community Treatment (ACT)
- Correctional facilities
- Work sites, foster care residences
- Home care
- Self-employed (advanced practice nurses)
- Primary care settings
- Academic settings
- Forensic settings
- Telehealth

- The delivery of mental health services through telecommunications technology removes time and distance barriers. The psychiatric–mental health nurse can utilize electronic communication such as telephone consultation, interactive video sessions, websites, faxing, e-mail, image transmission, research, and educational programs.

ANA Social Policy Statement

Nursing's Social Policy Statement (ANA, 2003) is a document that nurses can use as a framework for understanding the profession's relationships with society and its obligation to those who receive nursing care. Nursing is dynamic, not static, and reflects the changing nature of societal needs. Table 5–1 presents the ANA *Social Policy Statement* for the nursing profession.

Table 5–1. Selected Statements From *Nursing's Social Policy Statement*

Values and Assumptions	Humans manifest an essential unity of mind/body/spirit
	Human experience is contextually and culturally defined
	Health and illness are human experiences
	The presence of illness does not preclude health nor does optimal health preclude illness
Essential Features of Professional Nursing	Attention to the full range of human experiences and responses to health and illness without restriction to a problem-focused orientation
	Integration of objective data with knowledge gained from an understanding of the patient's or group's subjective experience
	Application of scientific knowledge to the processes of diagnosis and treatment
	Provision of a caring relationship that facilitates health and healing

Reprinted from American Nurses Association, *Nursing's social policy statement* (2nd. ed.), Washington, DC: American Nurses Publishing. © 2003 American Nurses Association. Reprinted with permission.

Patient-Centered Care

In today's managed care environment, it is imperative for nurses to work collaboratively with patients and families with a shared responsibility for assessing and treating healthcare problems and for promoting their own health and well-being. Issues of import to the development of shared responsibility between healthcare providers and patients include:

- Incorporating patient family values, beliefs, knowledge, and backgrounds into planning and delivery of care
- Communicating and sharing comprehensive information with patients
- Involving patients and families in patient-centered discussion of a unified care plan activities and anticipated outcomes
- Encouraging patients and families to participate in all aspects of their care and clinical decision-making
- Collaborating between policy and program development to facilitate quality care

Institute of Medicine Report

The Institute of Medicine (2001) published a landmark report, *Crossing the Quality Chasm in Health Care*, with specific recommendations for ensuring quality patient-centered care. This report defined patient-centered care as care that:

- Respects and is responsive to individual patient preferences, needs, and values
- Is available in many forms other than face-to-face contact, such as the Internet and telephone
- Makes the patient the source of control in his or her own care, and incorporates shared decision-making
- Provides patients with free access to their personal medical information
- Provides full clinical knowledge that is evidence-based and reflective of the best available scientific knowledge
- Ensures patient safety from injury caused by the healthcare system
- Maintains efficiency in terms of resources, energy, ideas, and patient time
- Equitably provides care for all patients regardless of ethnicity, geographic location, or socioeconomic status

SCOPE AND STANDARDS OF PSYCHIATRIC NURSING PRACTICE

The source of the scope and standards of professional nursing practice in psychiatric–mental health is the American Nurses Association (ANA), the International Society for Psychiatric Nursing (ISPN), and the American Psychiatric Nurses Association (APNA). In 2007, the American Nurses Association published the current *Psychiatric–Mental Health Nursing: Scope and Standards of Practice*, representing a consensus among the three professional groups.

Psychiatric–Mental Health Nursing: Scope and Standards of Practice delineates the scope and standards of clinical practice across clinical healthcare settings, incorporating a nursing process format at both basic and advanced practice levels to identify a competent, safe level of nursing care. The Standards of Professional Performance describes a competent level of professional role behaviors in professional psychiatric–mental health nursing practice. There are six standards of nursing practice, and nine standards of professional performance. **Standards 5E through 5G (prescriptive authority and treatment, psychotherapy, consultation) apply only to advanced practice nurses.**

Promotion of professional standards that support high-quality nursing care help to advance the purposes of the profession and the healthcare of the nation. Professional standards also have significance as a resource for peer review and performance appraisal processes, and are an important means of evaluating and improving care through quality improvement programs.

Professional Standards of Psychiatric Nursing Practice

Professional standards for psychiatric–mental health nursing are detailed in the ANA's *Psychiatric–Mental Health Nursing: Scope and Standards of Practice* (2007) on pages 29 to 55.

Standard 1. Assessment

The Psychiatric–Mental Health Registered Nurse collects comprehensive health data that are pertinent to the patient's health or situation.

Standard 2. Diagnosis

The Psychiatric–Mental Health Registered Nurse analyzes the assessment data to determine diagnoses or problems, including level of risk.

Standard 3. Outcome Identification

The Psychiatric–Mental Health Registered Nurse identifies expected outcomes individualized to the patient or to the situation.

Standard 4. Planning

The Psychiatric–Mental Health Registered Nurse develops a plan that prescribes strategies and alternatives to attain expected outcomes.

Standard 5. Implementation

The Psychiatric–Mental Health Registered Nurse implements the identified plan.

- *Standard 5A. Coordination of Care:* The Psychiatric–Mental Health Registered Nurse coordinates care delivery.
- *Standard 5B. Health Teaching and Health Promotion:* The Psychiatric–Mental Health Registered Nurse employs strategies to promote health and a safe environment.
- *Standard 5C. Milieu Therapy:* The Psychiatric–Mental Health Registered Nurse provides, structures, and maintains a safe and therapeutic environment in collaboration with patients, families, and other healthcare clinicians.
- *Standard 5D. Pharmacological, Biological, and Integrative Therapies:* The Psychiatric–Mental Health Registered Nurse incorporates knowledge of pharmacological, biological, and complementary interventions with applied clinical skills to restore the patient's health and prevent disability.
- *Standard 5E. Prescriptive Authority and Treatment:* The Psychiatric–Mental Health Advanced Practice Registered Nurse uses prescriptive authority, procedures, referrals, treatments, and therapies in accordance with state and federal laws and regulations.
- *Standard 5F. Psychotherapy:* The Psychiatric–Mental Health Advanced Practice Registered Nurse conducts individual, couples, group, and family psychotherapy using evidence-based psychotherapeutic frameworks and nurse–patient therapeutic relationships.
- *Standard 5G. Consultation:* The Psychiatric–Mental Health Advanced Practice Nurse provides consultation to influence the identified plan, enhance the abilities of other clinicians to provide services for patients, and effect change.

Standard 6. Evaluation

The Psychiatric–Mental Health Registered Nurse evaluates the patient's progress toward attainment of outcomes.

ANA Standards of Professional Performance

Standard 7. Quality of Practice

The Psychiatric–Mental Health Registered Nurse systematically enhances the quality and effectiveness of nursing practice.

Standard 8. Education

The Psychiatric–Mental Health Registered Nurse attains knowledge and competency that reflect current nursing practice.

Standard 9. Professional Practice Evaluation

The Psychiatric–Mental Health Registered Nurse evaluates one's own practice in relation to the professional practice standards and guidelines, relevant statutes, rules, and regulations.

Standard 10. Collegiality

The Psychiatric–Mental Health Registered Nurse interacts with and contributes to the professional development of peers and colleagues.

Standard 11. Collaboration

The Psychiatric–Mental Health Registered Nurse collaborates with patients, families, and others in the conduct of nursing practice.

Standard 12. Ethics

The Psychiatric–Mental Health Registered Nurse integrates ethical provision in all areas of practice.

Standard 13. Research

The Psychiatric–Mental Health Registered Nurse integrates research findings into practice.

Standard 14. Resource Utilization

The Psychiatric–Mental Health Registered Nurse considers factors related to safety, effectiveness, cost, and impact on practice in the planning and delivery of nursing services.

Standard 15. Leadership

The Psychiatric–Mental Health Registered Nurse provides leadership in the professional practice setting and the profession. (ANA, 2007)

ANA CODE OF ETHICS

ANA Code of Ethics With Interpretive Statements

The American Nurses Association's *Code of Ethics for Nurses With Interpretive Statements* (2001) consists of nine provisions or proclamations describing the principled behaviors and professional attributes expected of professional nurses (see Table 5–2). These ethical provisions require that nurses uphold each patient's right to self-determination and right to be treated with respect regardless of age, race, creed, type of illness, sexual orientation, and social status. This means that nurses should promote a healthcare environment that takes into account and respects the human values, cultural customs, and spiritual beliefs of their patients.

Nurses also should maintain ethical standards of personal conduct compatible with the expectations of the profession and public confidence in the integrity of professional nurses. Ethical standards take into consideration the following assumptions:
- Ethical concepts cannot be considered apart from the social contextual environment in which they occur.
- Factors of family, religious, and cultural standards and beliefs are important determinants of ethical standards.
- Expected socialized behaviors of the profession serve to influence the nurse's understanding of ethical behavior.

The values and obligations expressed in the ANA's Code of Ethics apply to all nurses in all roles and settings, "not only those involved in direct patient care, but also those involved in administration, education, and research" (ANA, 2001). Having a written professional code of ethics is particularly important at a time when the nation is undergoing fundamental changes in delivery of care that create important ethical dilemmas.

The ANA Code of Ethics provides a framework for ethical decision-making.

Table 5–2. Proclamations of ANA's Code of Ethics With Interpretive Statements

1   The nurse, in all professional relationships, practices with compassion and respect for the inherent dignity, worth, and uniqueness of every individual, unrestricted by considerations of social or economic status, personal attributes, or the nature of health problems.

2   The nurse's primary commitment is to the patient, whether an individual, family, group, or community.

3   The nurse promotes, advocates for, and strives to protect the health, safety, and rights of the patient.

4   The nurse is responsible and accountable for individual nursing practice and determines the appropriate delegation of tasks consistent with the nurse's obligation to provide optimum patient care.

Continued

Table 5-2. Proclamations of ANA's Code of Ethics With Interpretive Statements (cont.)

5   The nurse owes the same duties to self as to others, including the responsibility to preserve integrity and safety, to maintain competence, and to continue personal and professional growth.

6   The nurse participates in establishing, maintaining, and improving healthcare environments and conditions of employment conducive to the provision of quality health care and consistent with the values of the profession through individual and collective action.

7   The nurse participates in the advancement of the profession through contributions to practice, education, administration, and knowledge development.

8   The nurse collaborates with other health professionals and the public in promoting community, national, and international efforts to meet health needs.

9   The profession of nursing, as represented by associations and their members, is responsible for articulating nursing values, for maintaining the integrity of the profession and its practice, and for shaping social policy.

Reprinted from American Nurses Association, *Code of ethics for nurses with interpretive statements,* Washington, DC: American Nurses Publishing. © 2001 American Nurses Association. Reprinted with permission.

Theoretical Approaches to Ethics

Ethics is an area of study that examines a person's value beliefs, choices, and actions. Two prominent approaches provide guidelines for use in ethical decision-making.
- *Utilitarianism* (Teleology or Situational Ethics)
  - Focuses on the consequences of actions; the end justifies the means
  - Risk- or cost-benefit analysis is the basis for making ethical decisions
  - Ethical decisions reflect actions that would result in the greatest good for the largest number of people
- *Deontology*
  - Actions can be evaluated ethically in and of themselves as being intrinsically right or wrong
  - Ethical decisions should be based on duty and obligation to others, absolute moral rules and principles that are fixed and do not change

Key Concepts in Ethical Decision-Making

Ethical decision-making is based on professional values articulated in the ANA *Code of Ethics with Interpretative Statements.* Key concepts of ethical decision-making are based on:
- *Justice:* Fairness to everyone, sound reason, rightfulness of decisions and actions
- *Beneficence:* The duty to do good, not harm, to others

- *Nonmaleficence:* The duty to do no harm to others, and to protect from harm those who cannot do so for themselves (e.g., children, mentally incompetent persons, abused victims)
- *Fidelity:* The duty to be true and loyal to others
- *Autonomy:* The duty to protect the rights of a person to self-determination (i.e., to make decisions and take actions without external control)
- *Veracity:* The duty to tell the truth, and not to lie or deceive another

Ethical Dilemmas

An *ethical dilemma* is a situation in which a choice must be made between two or more potentially justifiable ethical choices. *Example:* Underinsured patients in managed care situations. Nurses can experience conflict between ethical positions held by their place of employment and personal values, religious or cultural beliefs. An ethical decision-making process involves the following:
- Collect, analyze, and interpret all relevant data, including the views of all stakeholders
- State the dilemma
- Consider all potential choices of action
- Make the decision; whenever possible, the patient's wishes should be followed, and ideally, it should be a collaborative decision

LEGAL ASPECTS OF PSYCHIATRIC NURSING PRACTICE

Protective Legal Rights

Both federal and state laws affect psychiatric–mental health nursing practice. Federal laws that protect the rights of mentally disabled individuals include:
- *Protection and Advocacy for Mentally Ill Individuals Act* (1986): Mandates that all states must designate an agency responsible for protecting the rights of mentally ill patients.
- *Americans with Disabilities Act* (ADA, 1990): Protects individuals with physical or mental disabilities from discrimination related to their disabilities and requires reasonable accommodations based on disability.
- *Patient Self-Determination Act* (1990): Protects the rights of mentally ill patients whose mental symptoms result in alternating periods of competence and incompetence; bipolar disorder is one example. Advance directives for mental health are written documents that specify how the patient wishes treatment decisions (e.g., medications, choice of hospital facility) to be made during episodic periods of incompetence.

Patient Rights

Psychiatric patients have specific and general rights. The specific rights can vary from state to state. Rights of institutionalized patients are established by the state statutes and vary greatly. Any time any of these rights are denied, there must be a sound reason and it must be documented. Denial of rights can never be punitive. In general, patients have the right to:

- Adequate, appropriate treatment, which includes
  - A humane psychological and physical environment
  - Qualified personnel to provide individualized care and individualized treatment plans
  - The right to be released if not dangerous
  - The right to aftercare

Some basic rights typically covered by statute are:
- Confidentiality
- Issues of involuntary detention
- To send and receive mail
- To consult with personal physician, attorney, or clergy
- Visitation, unless there are documented reasons for denial
- To use allowable (safe) personal possessions
- Privacy and private storage space
- Self-determination
- To refuse treatment or medication. All patients have the right to refuse medication, except for limited use during emergency situations or when they are court-ordered to take the medication
- To refuse psychosurgery or electroconvulsive therapy (ECT)
- To receive help from patient advocates
- Right to least-restrictive treatment environment refers to a balance between maintaining the highest level of patient freedom and providing appropriate behavioral emergency treatment.

Restraint and Seclusion

Restraining a patient's behavior, either physically or chemically with medication, is an *emergency form of treatment* reserved for behavioral situations in which the patient's symptom behavior justifies temporary restraint or seclusion to protect the patient from harming him- or herself or others. The Joint Commission (2008) provides very specific guidelines for implementing restraints:
1. Only to ensure the physical safety of the patient or other persons
2. When less restrictive interventions have been tried and are not successful
3. Only with the written order of a physician or healthcare provider. The written order must include a specific episode with identified start and end times.

Patients can be restrained temporarily for serious medical or behavioral symptoms. Examples of medical reasons for restraints include the patient's inability to cooperate with an essential physical treatment or device such as an IV, indwelling catheter, respirator, or dressing; or because of confusion or irrational thinking. Behavioral health reasons consist of severe behaviors that potentially could cause injury to self or others because of violent, aggressive, or acute agitation related to an emotional or behavioral disorder, or symptoms associated with acute drug use.

Regardless of the reason for the restraint or seclusion, the Joint Commission standards apply (The Joint Commission, 2008). Only the minimal amount of restraint necessary to ensure the safety of the patient and others, while promoting the patient's personal autonomy to the highest level possible, can be used. During the entire time of emergency treatment, physical assessment of the patient in behavioral seclusion or restraint must be documented in the chart at designated intervals, related to
- Signs of injury associated with the application of restraint or seclusion
- Nutrition/hydration

- Circulation and range of motion in the extremities
- Vital signs
- Hygiene and elimination
- Physical and psychological status and comfort
- Readiness of discontinuation of restraint or seclusion

Types of Restraint
- *Physical restraint* refers to any device, garment, or physical hold that restricts a person's voluntary movement and cannot be easily removed by the person.
- *Chemical restraint* refers to psychotropic medication given for the specific purpose of controlling behavior. Its therapeutic value lies in decreasing a patient's escalating anxiety and potential to harm self or others. When restrictive measures are necessary, nurses should document which less-restrictive measures were tried unsuccessfully, and specifically why the particular restrictive measure is necessary.

Federal Guidelines for Evaluation of Patients in Restraints or Seclusion
- CMS: Initial evaluation must be made within 1 hour by a licensed independent practitioner (LIP)
- Time restrictions in written orders for seclusion/restraints (renewal of orders is possible up to a maximum time of 24 hours, using the same time limit restrictions)
  - Adults: 4 hours
  - Adolescents (ages 9–17): 2 hours
  - Children (ages younger than 9): 1 hour

Documentation of care for the person in restraints or seclusion should include
- Rationale for the restraint or seclusion, including the patient's condition or symptoms and the less-restrictive alternatives and measures tried prior to restraint or seclusion use.
- Hourly face-to-face medical and behavioral evaluation, including a description of the behavior and interventions attempted.
- The patient's response to treatment interventions, and rationale for continued use of restraint or seclusion, if warranted.

Informed Consent

Informed consent is a communication issue as well as a legal and ethical one. All patients must have the capacity to understand the nature of the proposed treatment, receive adequate information to make an informed decision, and be presented with options to make an informed choice.

Informed consent is a matter of concern for patients with serious mental disorders. They often have more difficulty understanding a proposed treatment or have diminished capacity to fully comprehend its meaning to them because of cognitive processing symptoms associated with their mental disorder. For this reason, psychiatric–mental health nurses must be extremely attentive to the psychological and cognitive barriers these patients present to ensure accurate comprehension.

Informed Consent for Clinical Treatments
In most states, patients must give permission to be given psychotropic medications. The only exception is for emergency treatment in which the risk to health or life requires that treatment

be given immediately, and then only on a one-time basis. Patients must give informed consent to receive ECT and to participate in research studies.

Voluntarily hospitalized patients must sign consent for treatment at the time of admission. Involuntary patients cannot give informed consent. In this case, the guardian for the involuntary patient, court-appointed administrative treatment protocol, or an advance directive for mental health can override the patient's objection. Informed consent for psychiatric treatment requires that each person adequately understand the essential information needed to give informed consent. Informed consent also represents an ongoing communication process between nurses and patients receiving the medication or treatment, including the opportunity to ask questions and to have relevant provider contact information for further questions or dialogue. Information the patient needs to provide informed consent includes:
- The diagnosis and target symptoms for which the medication or treatment is being prescribed
- Trade and generic names of all medication
- The benefits/intended effects of the treatment or medication
- The risks and side effects of each medication or treatment
- Significant drug–drug, food–drug interactions
- Information regarding appropriate dosing and administration of medications
- The possible results of not taking the recommended medication as prescribed
- The possibility of needing to make changes in medication dosages based on the patient's condition
- Alternatives to the proposed medication or treatment
- A statement of the person's right to withdraw voluntary consent for medications or treatment at any time (unless the medication or treatment is mandated as part of court-ordered treatment or there is a significant change in the person's condition requiring one-time emergency treatment)
- If medication treatment is provided as a result of an emergency situation without obtaining the consent of the person, the nurse needs to document the emergency situation and the rationale for the one-time emergency use of a medication or treatment, and the time the medication was administered, in writing. Thereafter, informed consent must be obtained voluntarily from the patient for further administration of the medication or treatment.

Informed Consent for Research Studies
Informed consent also is needed for all research studies. Congress established Protection of Human Subjects in Biomedical and Behavioral Research legislation in 1974. The law requires a true informed consent by any individual before becoming a subject in a research project. Patients must sign and understand a written informed consent to participate in any research protocols. They can never unknowingly participate in research. Children under the age of 18 can give assent, but only a legally responsible adult can give official consent.

The informed consent process must provide information about:
- The nature and purpose of the research study
- The duration of the study
- How the data will be collected, used, and reported
- Any potential harm or discomfort that might reasonably be expected from the study
- Any known and potential consequences and side effects that may result from participation in the study
- The patient's right to stop participation in the study at any time without penalty

Personal Barriers to Informed Consent

Patient characteristics or situations that preclude an adequate understanding or comprehension of the information required to complete an informed consent process are considered personal barriers to informed consent. Examples include a patient's

- Cognitive deficits
- Primary language differences
- Level of literacy
- Fatigue
- Level of psychological stress

Documentation of the information given to the patient and the patient's consent should be included in the medical record.

Advance Directives for Mental Health

Some mental disorders present as episodic flare-ups with periods of unimpaired capacity in between (e.g., bipolar disorder). During a period of unimpaired capacity, the patient may legally initiate an advance directive for mental health care, which is designed to give specific written or oral instructions about treatment, and may appoint a power of attorney for heath care. The advance directive is a legal document providing specific instructions about such matters as where the patient should be hospitalized, treatment desires, and the name of the healthcare agent charged to make healthcare decisions in the event of the person's incapacity. This agent must follow the directions given by the patient in his or her period of competency.

Evaluation of Competency

Psychiatric–mental health nurses must understand the concept of competency because patients must be competent to give informed consent. Competence involves the patient's ability to

- Understand the information provided
- Reason the implications logically through to making a decision
- Appreciate the consequences of making one choice over another
- Clearly express a reasonable choice

Competency is not necessarily a fixed idea; incompetence can be episodic with some mental disorders. As in the case of bipolar disorder, or major depressive episodes, competence can be reestablished during remissions. A person under the influence of psychoactive drugs or severely stressed may not be competent at one point yet fully competent at another. Competency also is an issue in a court of law, where it is used to determine whether a person with mental illness is competent to proceed with trial, meaning able to aid his or her defense attorney and to understand the charges.

If a competency evaluation determines that a person is incompetent, an appropriate mental health provider has diagnosed a person to be physically and/or mentally unable to make a well-reasoned, deliberate, and knowledgeable healthcare decision. In this situation, a guardian or conservator is legally appointed to make healthcare decisions for the patient until such time as he or she is judged to be competent.

- *Guardianship/conservatorship* refers to a prescribed legal process in which a person or agency is appointed by the court to act on behalf of the disabled person. The guardian or conservator can make decisions on behalf of the patient, as well as provide informed consent for the identified patient when the patient is unable to do so. This person also has the authority over the individual's finances.

Legal Issues in Treating Minors

Only parents or legal guardians have the legal right to make treatment decisions for minors, unless they are emancipated. Minors are defined as all individuals under the age of 18 years. The authority of a parent can come to an end for minors upon the appointment by a court of a guardian for the minor, or through a legal process in which the adolescent requests a court to declare him or her emancipated. The Emancipation of Minors Act allows for a legal process in which a mature minor, demonstrating the ability and capacity to manage his or her own affairs and living independently of parents or guardian, may obtain the legal status and power to enter into valid legal contracts. There is some variation among the states to exact protocols, but in general, criteria for emancipation include one or more of the following:
- Marriage of the minor
- Enlistment of the minor as a member on active duty in the U.S. military
- Living independently and maintaining financial independence

Legal Rights of Minors
- *Confidentiality:* Parents have the legal right to review their child's record unless there is legal documentation that the court has terminated parental rights. At the beginning of treatment, this should be discussed with the minor and the parents, defining what information will be shared and what will be kept private. The minor also can authorize release of medical records.
- *Privilege:* Confidentiality relating to legal matters; parents usually hold the privilege to disclose or not to disclose in a court of law.
- *Exceptions to parents:* The therapist can refuse to allow parents to inspect the records when the minor is the victim of a crime or when there is a court-appointed guardian/custodian holding privilege.
- *No parental consent:* When the minor is 12 or older, presents good reason to not involve parents, and is mature enough to participate intelligently in outpatient treatment, parental consent need not be obtained. Clinical issues that can be treated without parental consent include help for substance abuse and prevention or treatment of pregnancy; when the child has been the alleged victim of incest or child abuse (including rape); and when the minor might be a serious threat, mentally or physically, to self without treatment.
- *Fees for treatment of a minor:* Parents are not held responsible for payment for treatment of their minor child when the parent has not been contacted and has not given consent.
- *Therapist responsibility:* Involve parents in treatment of a minor unless the therapist believes it is not in the best interest of the minor. The therapist must chart in the record if or when the parents were notified or, if not notified, why it was considered inappropriate to do so.

Custody
When parents divorce or die, the court establishes legal arrangements to provide for the care of minor children. The parent or caregiver who is awarded custody has the decision-making

responsibility regarding health care, education, and religious upbringing. There are different types of custody.

- *Joint custody:* Both parents hold physical and legal custody equally. Joint physical custody means that the child will physically live at both parent's homes with an equal amount of scheduled time spent at each parent's residence. Legal custody means that both parents are involved in making decisions and financial obligations.
- *Sole legal custody:* One parent has the right and responsibility to make the decisions relating to the health, education, and welfare of the child. The other parent generally is awarded defined visitation rights.
- *Joint legal custody:* Both parents have the right and responsibility to make the decisions relating to the health, education, and welfare of the child.
- *Sole physical custody:* The child resides with and under the supervision of one parent, subject to the court's power to order visitation.
- *Joint physical custody:* Both parents have significant periods of physical custody to assure a child of frequent and continuing contact with both parents.

LAWS AFFECTING PSYCHIATRIC NURSING PRACTICE

Common Types of Laws

- *Statutory law:* Statutory laws are found in federal and state legislated law. Laws drafted at the local level include city codes and regulations.
- *Common law:* Common laws involve negligence and malpractice. They evolve from previous legal decisions, which form a precedent over time.
- *Civil law:* A breach of civil law by nurses most frequently involves a violation of a patient's legal rights or a wrongful act that causes a patient injury. A tort is defined as a wrongful act committed against a person or his or her property that involves a violation of a patient's legal rights, or of a standard of care that causes patient injury. Intentional torts include assault and battery.
- *Negligence:* The commission or omission of an act that falls below the accepted standard of care. In a court of law, negligence is judged based on what a reasonable and prudent nurse would ordinarily do, or would not have done, in a similar situation.
- *Malpractice:* A type of negligence for which the nurse can be sued in court. To meet the criteria for malpractice in a court of law:
  - The duty was obligated to the patient because of the professional relationship.
  - There was a breach of duty in which the actions of the nurse violated this duty and/or failed to adhere to appropriate standards of care.
  - The breach of duty was the immediate cause of the resulting injury.
  - There were substantive damages or injury that resulted directly from the breach of duty.

  Clinical Examples: Failure to obtain informed consent, failure to report a change in the patient's condition, failure to take appropriate action to provide for a patient's safety.

Civil Commitment

- *Voluntary admission* to a hospital or treatment center begins with the written application of the patient, or patient's guardian in the case of a minor. The patient or patient's guardian can initiate discharge and the patient retains all civil rights. Voluntary patients who elect to leave the hospital against medical advice must sign a form indicating this is their intent.
- *Involuntary admission* does not originate with the patient, but is initiated by the hospital or court. Depending on individual state laws, the patient may lose some or none of their civil rights during the time of involuntary confinement. A petition for involuntary admission can be placed by a police officer, a psychiatrist, other designees appointed by the state, or the patient's family. Specific state mandates vary, but usually one or two physicians are required to medically certify that the patient is in need of involuntary confinement based on their examination of the patient's mental status. In some states, a psychiatric–mental health nurse clinician has this authority.
- *Civil commitment* laws involve legal processes leading to involuntary commitment. They are also used to determine the legal declaration of mental illness and provide guidelines for when a person can be placed in an inpatient setting without their consent. Civil commitment procedures allow states to involuntarily commit a patient to a mental health facility or hospital when the patient is unable to take care of him- or herself because of mental illness. Civil commitment laws vary from state to state, although commonly the criteria involve
  - Having a serious mental illness that creates a lack of insight about the need for hospitalization
  - Being an immediate danger to self or others due to a mental illness
  - Being unable to care for him/herself due to a mental illness

An initial confinement in a medical facility can be placed for up to 72 hours. If the individual is still considered a danger to self or others or is gravely disabled, he or she can be placed on an additional 14-day certification, but a court hearing must be held to uphold the confinement of individuals beyond this time. Patients are entitled to have their commitment reviewed every 6 months. These laws vary from state to state.

Insanity Defense for Mentally Ill Persons

Two types of insanity defenses are used for mentally ill patients who commit a criminal act: Not guilty by reason of insanity, or guilty but mentally ill. Successful defenses can result in treatment hospitalization in a state hospital rather than in a prison. The burden of proof is on the defense to determine if a person is competent to stand trial or engage in legal processes. The most frequently used legal standards to determine criminal responsibility are

- *McNaughten Rule:* The person lacks the mental capacity to understand that his or her actions were legally wrong, or is mentally unable to understand the physical nature or quality of his or her act.
- *Irresistible Impulse Test:* The mentally ill person was impulsively driven to commit the criminal action and could not control his or her actions due to lack of mental capacity, even if he or she knew the actions to be wrong.

CULTURALLY COMPETENT CARE

The *Surgeon General's Report on Mental Health: Culture, Race, Ethnicity* (U.S. Department of Health and Human Services, 2001) defines culture broadly as "a common heritage or set of beliefs, norms, and values" (p. 9). Cultural diversity finds expression in the patient's language; decision-making; food preferences; and ethnically influenced responses to stress, pain, sorrow, anger, bereavement, and the meaning of a mental illness.

Psychiatric–mental health nurses have a legal, ethical, and professional responsibility to respect, acknowledge, and incorporate cultural attitudes, beliefs, values, and behaviors into their clinical practice. Cultural and ethical values color the nurse's responses as well as those of the patient. Culture is a community concept that helps explain a person's worldview and provides significant resources and comfort to people in times of stress.

Concepts

Healthy People 2010 states that culturally competent health care is essential to eliminating health disparities. Common concepts related to culture include diversity, stereotyping, acculturation, and assimilation.

- *Diversity* refers to differences between cultures. Variation among members of the same culture is also the rule, rather than the exception. Factors such as urbanization, education, socioeconomic status, firsthand exposures, and religion all impact the variations found among people within the same culture.
- *Discrimination* is defined as "differences in care that emerge from biases and prejudice, stereotyping, and uncertainty in communication and clinical decision-making" (Institute of Medicine, 2002, p. 160).
- *Stereotyping* refers to over-simplified beliefs about a person or cultural group, often based on inaccurate data, and/or overgeneralizations (e.g., all mentally ill individuals are dangerous).
- *Ethnocentrism* refers to the belief that one's own culture is superior to all others.
- *Acculturation* refers to a socialization process in which a person from a different cultural group begins to learn and adopt the language and behavior patterns of the dominant culture as a result of firsthand contact.
- *Assimilation* refers to the adoption of the behavior patterns of the dominant culture such that the original ethnic identification disappears or is suppressed. It usually occurs over several generations.

In 2002, the Institute of Medicine reported that racial and ethnic minorities typically receive a lower quality of health care than non-minorities, even when patients' insurance status and income are matched. Federal level initiatives to improve access to care and to help eliminate health disparities among different sectors of the population are found through the Office of Minority Health in the document *Healthy People 2010*. This document identifies national priorities for the health care of the nation. Students are encouraged to become familiar with the *Healthy People 2010* document as it relates to cultural aspects of mental health and the health of the nation.

Cultural Competence

Cultural competence is defined as the "ability of individuals to establish effective interpersonal and working relationships that supersede cultural differences" (Institute of Medicine, 2002, p. 554). The Joint Commission mandates the use of a trained interpreter when necessary for patient–provider communication, with criteria published under Title VI of the Civil Rights Act.

When assessing preferences of patients from a different culture, the nurse should take into consideration:
- Explanatory models of illness
- Traditional healing processes
- Lifestyle issues
- Types of family support and decision-making in health situations
- Spiritual healing practices and rituals
- Cultural norms about illness and modesty
- Truth-telling and level of disclosure about serious or terminal illness
- Ritual and religious ceremonies at time of death (Arnold & Boggs, 2007).

PAIN MANAGEMENT

Standards in Pain Management

The Joint Commission's pain management standards (2002) require that every inpatient be routinely assessed for pain, that pain assessment be documented, and that pain be managed for each patient. Specifically, these standards call for healthcare providers to:
- Recognize the right of patients to appropriate assessment and management of their pain
- Screen for the existence of pain, and assess for pain in all patients
- Record the results of the assessment in a way that facilitates regular reassessment and follow-up
- Establish standards for regular monitoring and intervention
- Educate relevant providers in pain assessment and management
- Establish policies and procedures that support appropriate prescription or ordering of pain medications
- Ensure that pain does not interfere with participation in rehabilitation
- Ensure staff competency in pain management
- Establish policies that support appropriate prescription and ordering of pain medications
- Educate patients and their families about the importance of effective pain management
- Include patients' needs for symptom management in the discharge planning process
- Collect data to monitor the appropriateness and effectiveness of pain management (pain control performance improvement plan)

The American Pain Society (APS) has identified pain as the fifth vital sign that should be assessed with each evaluation of the standard vital signs (temperature, pulse, respiration, and blood pressure). The difference in pain evaluation is that because it is a subjective sign, only the patient can advise you of its existence and intensity, verbally and nonverbally. In assessing for pain, it is important to ask questions about:

- Onset and duration
- Location
- Character of the pain (sharp, dull, burning, persistent, changes with movement, direct or referred pain)
- Intensity, using a 0 to 10 numerical rating scale, with 0 being no pain and 10 being unbearable pain
- Personal beliefs about pain and its management, fears about disease progression or adverse side effects
- Exacerbating and relieving factors
- Responses to current and past treatment
- Patient's emotional state
- History of substance dependence (crossover tolerance)

The International Association for the Study of Pain (IASP, 2008) describes pain as a "biopsychosocial experience that has many components in addition to nociception. These include sensory, emotional, cognitive, developmental, behavioral, spiritual, and cultural components, all of which are known to influence pain perception and response." Pain is what the patient says it is. The experience of pain can be acute or chronic. Even when pain medication is essential to successful treatment, behavioral interventions can result in reduced pain intensity and improvement in physical and psychosocial functioning.

Although chronic pain is typically a less intense sensory experience for patients than acute pain, it can be very debilitating as a physical and psychological experience for both patients and their families. In addition to the physical aspects of pain, chronic pain can compromise quality of life, as well as personal and professional relationships. Pain issues can be exacerbated by other psychosocial and behavioral factors. McCaffery (2001) notes that pain can exacerbate or cause symptoms of anxiety and depression.

The treatment goals for managing pain are to reduce acute and chronic pain to its lowest possible level, to restore physical functioning by increasing activity levels, and to decrease the psychological impact of pain on the person. Comprehensive pain management that incorporates psychological and rehabilitative interventions, with or without pain medication, is the treatment of choice for individuals with chronic pain. Examples of therapies found to be of particular use in treating patients with chronic pain include cognitive therapy restructuring strategies and imagery.

Medication for Pain Control

If it is determined that a patient's pain level warrants medication, other decisions come into play. For mild to moderate pain, the patient may be started on a nonopioid analgesic given orally, for example, every 4 hours. Sometimes, an analgesic combined with behavioral interventions is sufficient to control lower levels of pain. If this intervention is not sufficient to control the pain, a low dose of a short-acting opioid may be started.

The use of opioids is often essential for moderate to severe pain management. The key to successful pain control with opioids is to "start low and go slow." If the pain is not controlled with lower doses, it may be necessary to titrate the dose upward with small increments until appropriate pain relief is achieved. People with chronic pain can also experience "breakthrough" pain, which occurs episodically as more severe pain. These pain spikes can occur with or without triggers, such as too much activity or added stress. When breakthrough pain occurs, rescue medications, which are faster-acting, can be used episodically.

Nurses need to become familiar with all drugs used for pain management, including duration of action, immediacy of effect, appropriate dosage, dosing intervals, and side effects. Other relevant information relates to the patient's previous response to pain medication, and the use of psychoactive drugs in the past.

Pain Management and Comorbidity

The management of pain in patients with a history of substance abuse or with a comorbid psychiatric disorder such as depression, anxiety disorders, somatization disorders, or PTSD may require extra care in dosing and monitoring. Chronic pain and psychiatric disorders can be reciprocally interactive; the chronic pain can deepen psychological symptoms, and the heightened emotional reactivity of the mental disorder can intensify the level of pain.

Although physical dependence and tolerance are expected physiological correlates of extended opioid therapy for pain, their emergence should not be considered addiction. Physical dependence on a prescribed controlled substance represents a physiologic neuro-adaptation to the drug. It is not addiction, but if the opioid is stopped abruptly, the person is likely to experience a withdrawal syndrome.

Patients with co-occurring substance dependence present a difficult problem. Patients with substance use disorders, even if in recovery, may need larger doses of opioid medications for pain relief than the general population because of cross-tolerance. Substance use problems in patients who need opioid analgesics for pain relief are not always self-evident. There are often few physical markers to identify patients who may be substance abusers or at risk prior to initiating opioid therapy. Yet these patients are entitled legally and ethically to receive comparable pain management to those without this co-occurring disorder. Use of screening instruments, a careful medication and substance use history, and monitoring medication compliance can alert the nurse to consider the possibility of addiction from pain medications in patients with comorbid substance use disorders. Clues to the possibility of addiction in patients seeking opioid medications include:

- Seeking medication from more than one provider or resource (e.g., dentists, emergency departments, multiple pain clinics or providers)
- Not taking the medication as prescribed (e.g., taking multiple doses or at irregular times)
- Requesting prescriptions earlier than scheduled, or frequent reporting of prescription loss
- Resisting recommended changes in drug choice or dosage despite clear evidence of adverse side effects from opioids
- Routinely use alcohol or illegal drugs
- Routinely use prescribed benzodiazepines

Patients with co-occurring substance use disorders need to be carefully monitored and counseled before and during treatment to prevent abuse of drugs they may legitimately need for effective pain management. Consultation with an expert, or team management of such patients, may be warranted.

Non-Pharmacologic Strategies for Pain Management

Non-pharmacologic strategies are used in combination with pharmacologic interventions to help patients self-manage their pain. Including family members in the individualized decision-making process regarding the types of treatment to be used empowers patients and helps ensure compliance. Cognitive models have proven quite useful in helping patients cope with chronic pain (Lebovits, 2007).

Guided imagery in which a person is taught to shift attention from his or her pain to an imagined pleasant scene (such as watching the sun set, being with a special friend or at the beach) can be relaxing and decrease the perception of pain. There is both a relaxing and a distracting component to this therapeutic strategy.

Self-hypnosis, biofeedback, and relaxation strategies are also used to alter perceptions of pain. These techniques are active strategies that help people to focus their mind in ways that can calm them and ease pain. Biofeedback is a methodology that allows individuals to learn to control muscle tension, heart rate, breathing, and temperature as a way of reducing anxiety and stress. Patients are able to reduce their autonomic arousal and consequently alter pain levels.

Pain Management for Children

In the small child, pain can manifest in the pitch, frequency, and duration of crying, changes in color, and body movements. The young child may be more emotional or irritable than usual. Changes in activity (e.g., listlessness or not playing) also can signify pain. Sometimes the child provides clues to pain location, or will respond with nodding or yes when asked specifically about pain in a body part. Once children are able to comprehend language, they can be shown pictures of faces indicating intensity of pain and asked which one they think matches their pain level. The Wong-Baker FACES scale can give the nurse an indication of the level of pain that a child is experiencing.

Anxiety and distress exacerbate discomfort and pain. Children can become sensitized over time to repeated procedures, causing anticipatory anxiety, which in turn can increase the perception of pain.

It is difficult for parents to see their children in pain, and children respond to their parents' concern. Intervention to help parents feel more comfortable and confident in coping with a child's pain is essential. Some simple things you can suggest to help parents help their young children requiring pain management:
- Let children know what to expect in simple terms, for example, the order of events for invasive or painful procedures (this should be done in a matter-of-fact but compassionate way, close to the time of the procedure).
- Adolescents may need more in-depth teaching and time to ask questions than younger children.
- Assure the child that you will be with him or her.
- Don't tell the child it won't hurt if it will.
- Touch and being held are comforting to the child.
- Light massage, back rubs, and hand-holding help reduce a child's tension.

For older children, guided imagery, relaxation exercises, meditation, Reiki, acupuncture, and the cognitive therapy interventions described above can be helpful.

Pain Management in Adults With Cognitive Impairments

Adults with cognitive impairments often cannot articulate their pain. Instead they demonstrate pain nonverbally through facial grimacing or wincing, bracing, rubbing, agitation and restlessness. Often changes in typical behaviors are the first indicators. Finding the cause of the pain is the first priority. Relaxation techniques, music, and touch may also be helpful in reducing pain intensity and pain perception. Prayer, particularly those that are familiar from an earlier time, can relax patients with cognitive impairments who are spiritually inclined. Since patients who are older are more likely to experience negative side effects from pain medications, they will need to be monitored more closely.

RESOURCES FOR CONTINUING CARE

Interdisciplinary Collaboration

Gardner (2005) defines collaboration as "a process and an outcome in which shared interest or conflict that cannot be addressed by any single individual is addressed by key stakeholders." A collaborative outcome involves the development of integrative solutions that go beyond an individual vision to a productive resolution that could not be accomplished by any single person or organization. Interdisciplinary collaborative practices bring together multiple providers to achieve objectives aimed at meeting the mental health needs of patients and their families. Building collaborative relationships among the psychiatrist, clinical specialist or nurse practitioner, social worker, occupational therapist, recreational therapist, case manager, and so on, involved with a patient's care in face-to-face meetings enhances and extends care provision. All can contribute to identifying and monitoring safe, quality care for patients with mental illness. Collaborative discussions can include developing and sharing comprehensive treatment plans, making treatment decisions, resolving patient issues, setting treatment goals, and coordinating care within a cooperative, integrated framework. External collaborations can help hospitals and clinical agencies share information and resources with the community and important supporters of mental health such as religious leaders and traditional healers.

Gardner lists 10 ideas the nurse can use to become an effective collaborator with other interdisciplinary healthcare providers:
1. Know thyself. Many realities exist simultaneously. Each person's reality is based on self-developed perceptions. Requisite to trusting self and others is in knowing your own mental model (biases, values, and goals).
2. Learn to value and manage diversity. Differences are essential assets for effective collaborative processes and outcomes.
3. Develop constructive conflict resolution skills. In the collaborative paradigm, conflict is viewed as natural and as an opportunity to deepen understanding and agreement.
4. Use your power to create win-win situations The sharing of power and the recognition of one's own power base is part of effective collaboration.

5. Master interpersonal and process skills. Clinical competence, cooperation, and flexibility are the most frequently identified attributes important to effective collaborative practice.
6. Recognize that collaboration is a journey. The skills and knowledge needed for effective collaboration take time and practice. Conflict resolution, clinical excellence, appreciative inquiry, and knowledge of group process are all skills that can be improved throughout one's lifetime.
7. Leverage all multidisciplinary forums. Being present both physically and mentally in team forums can provide an opportunity to assess how and when to offer collaborative communications for partnership-building.
8. Appreciate that collaboration can occur spontaneously. Collaboration is a mutually established condition that can happen spontaneously if the right factors are in place.
9. Balance autonomy and unity in collaborative relationships. Learn from your collaborative successes and failures. Becoming part of an exclusive team can be as bad as working in isolation. Be willing to seek feedback and admit mistakes. Be reflective, willing to seek feedback, and admit mistakes for dynamic balance.
10. Remember that collaboration is not required for all decisions. Collaboration is not a panacea, nor is it needed in all situations.

Discharge Planning

Discharge planning is a patient-centered, interdisciplinary process that helps individuals with mental illness receive the adjunctive mental health care and/or case management they may need once discharged from the hospital. Discharge planning and teaching should begin with the patient's admission. The discharge plan should relate to the initial assessment of the patient's potential needs identified on admission to the inpatient setting. In addition to bearing in mind the patient's specific needs post-discharge, individualized discharge planning should consider

- Patient's physical, mental, cognitive, economic, and emotional strengths and abilities
- Patient's functional status
- Patient's support system and its availability
- Whether the patient needs post-hospital services and, if so, whether these services are available, and who will provide them
- Available community resources and public benefits, including financial assistance

Effective discharge planning requires ongoing collaboration among the patient, patient's family, and the interdisciplinary team in making informed decisions

For maximum effectiveness, discharge plans should be written and orally conveyed to the patient and patient's family. Written instructions should be clear, simple, and easy to understand. Each discharge plan contains common elements, as well as others tailored to the individualized needs of the patient. For example, discharge plans should summarize details about:

- Early signs of relapse and risky behaviors that can lead to relapse
- Medical and psychological strategies for handling early warning signs, including whom to contact if reemergence of symptoms is suspected
- Details of medication adherence, including dosage, treatment effects, and potential side effects
- An individualized recovery plan including bio-psychosocial treatments, informal and formal community-based support systems
- Referrals for case management and other essential social and financial supports

- The patient and family caregivers should be given provider contact phone numbers, and should be provided with emergency contact numbers

Service providers, case managers, and other agencies involved in the ongoing care of the patient should be contacted. A discharge summary and follow-up actions should be clearly spelled out in writing to all involved professionals (with the patient's written permission). Some communication, general or specific about patient needs, may need to be shared with primary providers.

Recovery Plans

A recovery model of mental illness takes a holistic view of a person with a serious mental illness, considering him or her from a strengths perspective. Based on the premise that people diagnosed with mental illness can function effectively in the community, the model proposes that even individuals with serious mental illness should take an active role in their own care. A recovery model focuses on helping people live in the community as productive citizens leading satisfying lives despite having a mental disability. Fundamental characteristics of a recovery model include:
- Self-determination and self-advocacy
- Hope and empowerment
- Viewing relapse as a temporary setback, with continued expectations of personal success
- Resiliency drawn from personal strengths, personalized support systems, and ongoing education about each person's clinical picture.

Wellness recovery action plans (WRAP) represent a person's road map for recovery. Each plan is individualized to reflect a person's needs, preferences, values, and culture. The plan includes personally defined goals, realistic objectives, and a strength-based orientation, with services and interventions needed for success clearly identified.

Although recovery models support self-determination and WRAP is driven and managed by the person who is receiving services, WRAP should identify and embrace the support of other people and services who can help consumers with mental illness achieve personal goals. Key elements of WRAP include:
- Developing a wellness tool box
- Creating a daily maintenance plan
- Identifying triggers and an action plan
- Identifying early warning signs and an action plan
- Planning for a crisis and the time after a crisis

Case Management

Because psychiatric and substance abuse disorders tend to be persistent and recurrent, many people with serious mental illnesses or chronic substance abuse problems require a continuous and integrated approach of assessment and treatment to function effectively, and to maintain self-sufficiency in the community. *Case management* is a unique form of treatment management in which a psychiatric nurse provides ongoing management support to vulnerable individuals with mental illnesses and/or their family and works with community agencies to ensure high quality coordination of care. Specific activities can include:
- Planning and coordination of treatment services in home and community environments

- Referring and linking to community services, including medical, educational, financial, social, vocational, and other rehabilitative resources
- Providing crisis intervention supports needed for immediate problem resolution
- Educating the patient and parent to improve daily functioning and self-sufficiency
- Assisting in the identification, planning, coordination, and implementation of mental health treatments as part of a multidisciplinary health team

REGULATORY GUIDELINES AFFECTING PSYCHIATRIC NURSING PRACTICE

Accreditation Process

Accreditation is a voluntary process through which national government and nongovernment accrediting bodies grant recognition to designated healthcare institutions that meet defined quality and safety standards in the care of patients and organizational management. Accreditation provides solid, consistent structural guidelines for professional development of staff and accountability for quality care. Accreditation processes are designed to encourage continuous improvement in patient care processes and outcomes, improve the management of healthcare services, and provide recognition for excellence in provision of safe, effective healthcare services. Reimbursement by governmental agencies such as Medicare, third-party payers, and vendors requires accreditation approval. Key inpatient organizational accreditation bodies include the Joint Commission, Health Insurance Portability and Accountability Act (HIPAA), Center for Medicare and Medicaid Services (CMS), and the Commission on Accreditation of Rehabilitation Facilities (CARF).

The Joint Commission

The Joint Commission, formerly known as the Joint Commission on Accreditation of Health Care Organizations, is the oldest and largest national healthcare accrediting body in the United States. The Joint Commission is committed to improving the quality and safety of patient care in inpatient healthcare organizations. The Joint Commission standards and performance measurements, which are reasonable expectations and able to be surveyed, provide a standardized objective evaluation process for healthcare organizations. These standards emphasize providing quality care to patients in safe healthcare environments. The 2009 standards draft for behavioral health is retrievable from http://www.jointcommission.org/Standards/SII/sii_bhc.htm.

The Joint Commission's website states:

> The mission of The Joint Commission is to continuously improve the safety and quality of care provided to the public through the provision of health care accreditation and related services that support performance improvement in health care organizations.

Key Regulatory Agencies for Outpatient Services

National Committee for Quality Assurance (NCQA) refers to a private, nonprofit agency that is the leader in health maintenance organization (HMO) accreditation. This agency provides information to employers, federal and state agencies, and consumers to assist them in selecting among competing health plans. This organization focuses on accreditation and performance measures related to access and service.

Health Plan Employer Data and Information Set (HEDIS) refers to the interactive tool implemented by NCQA and used by more than 90% of America's health plans to measure performance on important dimensions of care and service. NCQA's Health Plan Report Card is a written compilation of clinical quality, member satisfaction, and comprehensive evaluation of key systems and processes.

Center for Medicare and Medicaid Services (CMS) is the federal agency that administers the Medicare, Medicaid, and Child Health Insurance Programs. Medicare is a federal health insurance program providing coverage for persons 65 years and older and persons younger than 65 with long-term disabilities. *Medicaid* is a jointly funded state-federal health insurance program for eligible low-income persons. Certain requirements apply, such as age, disability, pregnancy, or blindness. People applying for Medicaid must meet other requirements related to financial resources and citizenship or legal residency. Coverage for Medicaid varies by state and is subject to federal requirements.

HIPAA Regulations

HIPAA is an acronym for the Health Insurance Portability and Accountability Act. This federal law, which went into effect in April 2003, places new requirements on the use of a patient's "protected health information" by covered entities such as individual healthcare providers, hospitals, nursing homes, clinics, mental health centers, and researchers. HIPAA defines protected health information (PHI) as any identifiable health information, including the name and contact information, that is or can reasonably be linked to an individual. Release of such information is prohibited unless it is explicitly allowed by the privacy rule or the patient gives written consent. HIPAA:
- Defines who may see or use health information, and what they can do with it
- Limits uses and disclosures of health information to the minimum amount of necessary information needed for care
- Establishes broad new patient rights related to seeing and asking for corrections of their own health information

Protected health information (PHI) includes all identifiable patient information related to past, present, or future physical or mental health needs, treatment provision, or payment for the provision of mental health care of patients. For example, PHI would include who provided the care, what type of care was provided, where the care was given, when the care was provided, and the rationale for providing the care. This information can only be transmitted when the patient, or someone legally acting on the patient's behalf, provides written permission to do so.
   Potential sources of PHI appear in the form of:
- Written information (e.g., charts, letters, notes, reports)

- Oral communication (e.g., phone calls, meetings, informal conversations)
- Computerized and electronic communication (e.g., e-mail, computer records, faxes, voicemail, PDA or BlackBerry® entries)

Privacy maintenance of PHI in patient records requires that nurses
- Use and do not share computer passwords
- Keep records behind locked doors in locked file cabinets
- Limit access to
  - Workspace where health information is stored or used
  - Printers and fax machines where health information is printed
  - Only those professionals who need the information for a specific function or health-related care task

With *written* consent, the advanced practice nurse can disclose PHI to another professional or covered entity in such situations as:
- A third-party insurance company for reimbursement purposes
- For limited tasks (e.g., compliance, quality improvement, or peer review)
- Referral for treatment or report to a primary care physician
- Coordination of care or consultation between healthcare providers when both have a relationship with a patient

Allowable HIPAA Disclosures
Disclosures are allowed by HIPAA only:
- For judicial and administrative proceedings in response to a written order of the court or an administrative tribunal, or in response to subpoena, discovery request, or "other lawful process." The requester or healthcare provider must give notice to the patient or get a protective order from the court first.
- To avert serious threat to the health or safety of a person or the public. Disclosures must be only to the person reasonably able to prevent or lessen the threat, or only when it is necessary for law enforcement personnel to identify or apprehend an individual.

Privileged communication does not fall under HIPAA supervision. It refers exclusively to court proceedings, and is designed to protect the provider from having to reveal in court a patient's communication without the patient's written permission. This means that the nurse cannot be called to testify as a witness in a court procedure without the patient's written permission to release information about him- or herself.

ISSUES RELATED TO REIMBURSEMENT OF MENTAL HEALTH SERVICES

Carve-Outs

Mental healthcare services for both adults and children are increasingly being controlled financially by managed behavioral health organizations. Reimbursement for mental health and substance abuse services are handled as "*carve-outs,*" meaning that insurance payments are financially separated from those provided for other clinical services, and are managed under a separate contract. Carve-outs have separate provider networks. These carve-outs were designed as a way to restrict the potential high costs of long-term psychotherapy and extended hospital stays associated with some forms of mental illness. Most carve-out options have separate, lower annual lifetime limits on care per person and per episode.

Medicaid and Medicare also impose financial restrictions on long-term care of mental disorders. The impact of managed care on mental healthcare delivery has been to foster short-term treatment and to cut the cost of mental health services. Ideally, these cost-cutting measures will not lower the quality of care or prevent access to necessary treatment.

Managed Care

Managed care refers to a broad category of health insurance plans designed to provide individuals and families with a range of healthcare services at a reduced cost. The goal of managed care services for mental health and substance dependence disorders is to provide the best, individualized, cost-effective care to patients.

Managed care plans differ in cost, degree of provider choice, and flexibility of service area. Primary forms of managed care consist of health maintenance organizations (HMO), point of service plans (POS), and preferred provider organizations (PPO).

Health maintenance organizations (HMO) are closed healthcare systems in which the primary care physician coordinates the patient's specialty care and most mental health services require a primary care provider referral or direct authorization from the HMO carve-out management company. While the most restrictive, HMO coverage is usually the least costly. As an HMO subscriber, a person pays a monthly premium with a small co-pay for primary or specialty care, and all necessary care is provided through the HMO contracted or group practice physicians and other healthcare providers. There are exceptions for emergency treatment or medically necessary treatment not obtainable through the HMO, with HMO approval. Components of major HMOs include:
- *Utilization review:* Cases are reviewed to ensure appropriate length of stay, medical necessity, and suitable level of care.
- *Case authorization and referral:* Patients must receive authorization for mental health treatment. The managed care organization oversees the mental health care, and monitors level of treatment for the behavioral healthcare program.
- *Quality assurance/improvement:* Patients are followed from intake through the treatment process with treatment plans required for authorization of further treatment. The purpose of this monitoring and follow-up is to ensure that the benefit dollar is spent in providing quality care throughout the mandated mental healthcare program.

Point of service plans (POS) offer subscribers a choice to select an HMO, a PPO, or an out-of-network provider. Depending on the choice of provider (e.g., out of network), the person can pay a larger share of the cost and typically has higher deductibles. POS plans offer the most flexibility for people traveling beyond the designated service area and needing care.

Preferred provider organizations (PPO) are service plans in which the insurance organization contracts with care providers who then are reimbursed at a discounted service rate for their professional services. This type of plan usually has higher monthly premiums, and an annual deductible must be met before coverage begins.

Advanced practice nurses must be nationally certified in their specialty, hold an active professional RN license, and apply for a Universal Provider Identification number (UPIN) to be accepted as an HMO or PPO provider. The UPIN is a permanent identifying number assigned to a qualified mental health provider.

Alternative Funding

Serious disparities still exist in accessing public mental health services, particularly for minority and migrant populations and illegal immigrants. Alternative funding for mental health priorities is essential for the many citizens who are not covered by Medicaid and dedicated state or locally funded public mental health programs. Some of the alternative funding for services used to maintain individuals with mental illness in the community include wraparound services for children and block grant funds providing the uninsured with mental health services. Other sources include public housing programs or waivers, which can help individuals with mental illness achieve enough economic self-sufficiency to survive in the community. This type of assistance is essential as it is estimated that more than 30% of homeless individuals have a serious mental disorder. The juvenile justice system serves as an alternative funding source for the many children who receive initial mental health treatment within the legal system.

Social security disability insurance (SSDI) and supplemental security (SSI) funds may be available to individuals with documented psychiatric problems who are unable to survive financially in the community. Migrant health centers can provide mental health care for individuals who qualify. More recently, mental health courts in several states are using forced treatment for offenders with a mental illness as an option in lieu of prosecution or as a condition for reduced charges. Head Start programs are used to provide comprehensive developmental services for preschool children and their parents. Church-affiliated mental health services are offered at a reduced rate or sliding scale (e.g., Ephesians for drug abuse and comorbid mental health problems).

Community Advocacy Resources

Community resources for mental health vary from state to state and from county to county within a state. Information about specific public and nonprofit mental health services can be found on county government websites. Most counties have mental health and alcohol/drug abuse advisory committees composed of providers, consumers, lawyers, religious, school, and law enforcement representatives. These advisory boards advocate for the mentally ill, advise the county government on community needs (e.g., third-shift crisis center coverage), and make recommendations for enhancement of the public mental health system and local community resources. Support groups, such as the National Alliance on Mental Illness (NAMI), On Our Own, Sante Group, Survivors of Suicide, and so on are available in the community. These groups are part of a network of support that helps maintain people in need of mental health services in the community.

Wrap-around services is a form of community-based, intensive mental health services available to families with children and adolescents with multiple psychological and social issues. The program is designed to provide families with a variety of supports to prevent the need for more restrictive levels of care. The purpose of providing these home- and school-based supports is to enhance the capacity of families to cope with difficult issues in both home and school settings. With wrap-around services, the juvenile and his or her family are considered important parts of the treatment team.

An increasing number of communities are developing *ACT teams (Assertive Community Treatment)* to reduce recidivism with chronically and persistently mentally ill patients. The ACT service delivery model provides comprehensive, immediate treatment for individuals with serious and persistent mental illness within their home environment. These services are available to mentally ill individuals and their families 24 hours a day, 7 days a week. The ACT multidisciplinary team acts as a unit and works collaboratively to provide treatment, rehabilitation, and support services to identified individuals in need of mental health services. The ACT team is available to these individuals whenever and wherever needed. According to NAMI, 6 states have statewide ACT programs, and 19 have at least one ACT pilot program.

Head Start preschool programs were developed to provide comprehensive developmental and social services for low-income preschool children aged 3 to 5 years. The purpose of Head Start programs is to stimulate the social and cognitive development of children through provision of health, nutrition, and social services to build self-esteem and promote school readiness. This type of community support is available in most states.

Many communities provide temporary shelters for homeless mentally ill individuals, although the need far exceeds availability. The public mental health system has case management capabilities for qualified individuals to help serious and chronically mentally ill individuals navigate the public health and social system. Crisis and detox centers exist in most larger and urban communities. Depending on the jurisdiction and available funding, these can operate on a 24-hour basis. Again, the need exceeds availability.

Grassroots peer support efforts are a growing community resource. NAMI is a self-help, support, and advocacy organization of people with severe mental illnesses and their families and friends. Peer-to-peer counseling, recovery support groups led by people living with mental illness, education, and support for family members are offered by NAMI (National Alliance for Mental Illness) and patient advocacy groups such as On Our Own.

REFERENCES

American Association of Colleges of Nursing. (2008). *The essentials of baccalaureate education for professional nursing practice.* Retrieved February 3, 2009, from www.aacn.nche.edu/Education/bacessn.htm

American Nurses Association. (2001). *Code of ethics for nurses with interpretative statements.* Washington, DC: American Nurses Publishing.

American Nurses Association. (2003). *Nursing's social policy statement* (2nd ed.). Washington, DC: American Nurses Publishing.

American Nurses Association. (2004). *Nursing: Scope and standards of practice.* Washington, DC: American Nurses Publishing.

American Nurses Association. (2007). *Psychiatric–mental health nursing: Scope and standards of practice.* Silver Spring, MD: Author.

American Nursing Credentialing Center. (2008). *2008 General testing and renewal handbook.* Silver Spring, MD: Author. Available at http://www.nursecredentialing.org/Certification/CertificationRenewal/GeneralTestingandRenewalHandbook.aspx

Arnold, E., & Boggs, K. (2007). *Interpersonal relationships: Communication skills for nurses* (5th ed.). St. Louis, MO: Elsevier Health Sciences.

Barloon, L. (2000). Legal aspects of psychiatric nursing. *Nursing clinics of North America, 38*(1), 9–19.

Copeland, M. E. (2007). *About WRAP [Wellness Recovery Action Plan].* Retrieved February 16, 2009, from http://www.mentalhealthrecovery.com/aboutwrap.php

Gardner, D. (2005). Ten lessons in collaboration. *Online Journal of Issues in Nursing, 10*(1). Retrieved February 3, 2009, from www.nursingworld.org/MainMenuCategories/ANAMarketplace/ANAPeriodicals/OJIN/TableofContents/Volume102005/No1Jan05/tpc26_116008.aspx

Gureje, O., Von Korff, M., Simon, G. E., & Gater, R. (1998). Persistent pain and well-being: A World Health Organization study in primary care. *Journal of the American Medical Association, 280,* 147–151.

Institute of Medicine. (2001). *Crossing the quality chasm: A new health system for the 21st century.* Washington, DC: The National Academy Press. Available at http://www.nap.edu/books/0309072808/html/

Institute of Medicine. (B. D. Smedley, A. Y. Stith, & A. R. Nelson, Eds.). (2002). *Unequal treatment: Confronting racial and ethnic disparities in health care.* Washington, DC: The National Academies Press.

The International Association for the Study of Pain. (2008). *Outline curriculum on pain for schools of nursing* (2nd ed.). Retrieved February 3, 2009, from http://www.iasp-pain.org/AM/Template.cfm?Section=Nursing&Template=/CM/HTMLDisplay.cfm&ContentID=2320

The Joint Commission on Accreditation of Health Care Organizations. (2002). *New JCAHO pain care treatment standards.* Retrieved February 3, 2009, from http://www.ipcaz.org/pages/new.html

The Joint Commission. (2008). *Restraint and seclusion standards.* Retrieved February 10, 2009, from http://www.jointcommission.org/AccreditationPrograms/BehavioralHealthCare/Standards/09_FAQs/PC/Restraint+_Seclusion.htm

Lebovits, A. (2007). Cognitive-behavioral approaches to chronic pain. *Primary Psychiatry, 14*(9), 48–54.

McCaffery, M. (1999). Assessing pain in a confused, nonverbal patient. *Nursing, 99*(7), 18.

McCaffrey, M. (2001). Overcoming barriers to pain management. *Nursing, 31*(4), 18.

McCaffery, M., & Pasero, C. (2001). Assessment and treatment of patients with mental illness: Implanting the JCAHO pain management standards. *American Journal of Nursing, 101*(7), 69.

National Council of State Boards of Nursing. (2008). *Boards of nursing.* Retrieved September 5, 2008, from https://www.ncsbn.org/boards.htm

Sparacino, P. S. A. (2005). The clinical nurse specialist. In A. B. Hamric, J. A. Spross, & C. M. Hanson (Eds.), *Advanced practice nursing: An integrative approach* (3rd ed., pp. 415–446). St. Louis, MO: Elsevier.

U.S. Department of Health and Human Services. (2001). *Mental health, culture, race, ethnicity supplement to mental health: Report of the Surgeon General.* Washington, DC: Author.

Vuckovich, P. (2003). Psychiatric advance directives. *Journal of the American Psychiatric Nurses Association, 9*(2), 55–59.

Wysoker, A. (2003). HIPAA and psychiatric nurses. *Journal of the American Psychiatric Nurses Association, 9*(5), 173–175.

Basic and Applied Science:
The Neuroscience of Mental Disorders

Karan Kverno, PhD, PMHNP-BC, PMHCNS-BC

ANATOMY AND PHYSIOLOGY THROUGH THE LIFE SPAN

In this chapter, we will examine the anatomy (structure) and physiology (function) of the nervous system, as well as major theories regarding the disruption of normal physiological functioning (pathophysiology) in selected mental disorders.

Physical Development

At birth, infants normally display characteristic primitive reflexes that include grasping, rooting, sucking, startle (moro), and Babinski reflex (toes spread when sole of foot is touched). The Babinski reflex disappears by about 1 year; the others, by about 4 months. By around 2 weeks of age, an infant prefers the mother's voice and has the ability to discriminate colors, smells, and tastes. Although development proceeds a bit differently for each individual, on average, other physical milestones include: balancing the head (4 months); sitting unsupported (6 months); pulling to feet (10 months); walking and grasping small objects (12–16 months); running (2 years); jumping, dancing, and drawing or copying simple objects (3 years); skipping (age 5); and riding a bike (6 years). The average age of puberty for girls is from 10 to 14 years, with menarche around 11 years; puberty for boys is from 10½ to 17½ years. At puberty, most individuals have a growth spurt and develop secondary sex characteristics. With aging, we expect to see a decline in most physical systems (Table 6–1). In certain neurodegenerative disorders, such as dementia, the primitive reflexes may return.

Table 6-1. Examples of Changes in Physical Systems With Aging

Physical Systems	Changes with Aging
Neurological	• Decreases in neurons and some neurotransmitters • Brain becomes smaller and lighter • Vision and hearing loss • Continued ability to form new synapses
Endocrine	• Changes in production of most hormones, change in function may not occur
Respiratory	• Decline in respiratory muscle strength and control of breathing
Cardiovascular	• Heart and blood vessels stiffen • Cardiac output declines • Decreased ability of heart and vessels to stress
Gastrointestinal	• Liver, gallbladder, and pancreas continue to function well in the elderly • Decreased hepatic blood flow may decrease drug clearance
Genitourinary	• Decreased size of kidneys • Decreased renal blood flow • Creatinine clearance declines • Erectile dysfunction in approximately 67% by age 70 (Stahl, 2008)
Musculoskeletal	• Decline in muscle mass with increasing weakness • Bone loss
Integumentary	• Increased dryness • Increased thinning and decreased elasticity • Wrinkles, dryness, and age spots from excessive sunlight
Hematologic	• Decreased ability of bone marrow to produce rapid increases in red blood cells with blood loss.

Brain Development

At birth, infants weigh an average of only 7 pounds, yet their head size is approximately one-third the size of their entire body. Even though the brain is relatively large compared to the body, it has not finished developing. With the help of glial cells and growth factors, neurons continue to migrate to their terminal sites within the frontal lobes, making connections with other neurons and laying down the structures that will guide executive functioning and self-regulation. Not until the late teens or early twenties is the development of the brain (and personality) complete. Throughout our lives, synapses are modified, solidifying memories or causing them to be forgotten. New neurons continue to be created in the area of the brain involved in consolidating long-term memories. Terms such as *neuroadaptation* and *neuroplasticity* describe the dynamic relationship between nature and nurture—between the brain and the environment.

NEUROANATOMY AND NEUROPHYSIOLOGY

The objectives of learning basic neuroanatomy and neurophysiology include gaining an ability to identify basic structures and functions within the nervous system, identifying neurotransmitter systems that are involved in psychiatric symptoms and disorders, and understanding the rationale for selected psychopharmacological interventions.

Organization of the Nervous System

The brain, brain stem, and spinal cord are the major structures of the central nervous system (CNS). The remainder of the nervous system is called the peripheral nervous system (PNS). The PNS is divided into the somatic branch that is involved in voluntary motor movement, and the autonomic branch (ANS) that controls the internal organs, blood vessels, and glands. The ANS is further divided into the sympathetic and parasympathetic branches. The activation of the sympathetic branch results in increased heart rate, respiration, blood pressure, and energy mobilization, and decreased digestive and reproductive functions. The parasympathetic branch of the nervous system serves more homeostatic functions by maintaining heart rate, respiratory, metabolic, and digestive functions under normal conditions.

The Brain

The brain weighs approximately 3 pounds, has several billion neurons, and has tens of billions of neuronal interconnections. The brain can be divided into three basic components: the cerebrum, the cerebellum, and the brain stem. The cerebrum is the outer- and upper-most part of the brain. Four major lobes are represented bilaterally, connected by a band of axons called the *corpus callosum*. In the majority of people, even those with left-hand dominance, verbal language functions are primarily represented in the left hemisphere, and nonverbal functions are primarily represented in the right hemisphere. Ascending and descending pathways carry information between the brain and spinal cord. The descending pathways traveling from the cortex to the spinal cord (corticospinal) cross to the opposite side in the brain stem. Thus an injury to the left frontal area of the brain may affect motor functioning on the right side of the body. By knowing the basic functions of the major lobes and structures, we can understand many of the behaviors and symptoms of psychiatric disorders. Descriptive terms referring to problems with higher level cognitive functioning are listed in Box 6–1.

Functions of the *frontal lobes* include motor control, executive functioning, working memory, and personality. Broca's area is the part of the motor cortex involved in the production of speech. Damage to this area can result in difficulty speaking and is referred to as *Broca's* (or nonfluent) *aphasia*. The foremost parts of the frontal cortex ("prefrontal cortex") are responsible for three major functions: 1) executive functioning, 2) working memory, and 3) personality. *Executive functioning* refers to decision-making, planning, organization, and impulse control. *Working memory* refers to an attentional system that can hold and manipulate information until it is transferred into long-term storage. Many of the psychiatric disorders (e.g., attention deficit-hyperactivity disorder, depression, schizophrenia) are characterized by deficits in executive and working memory functioning. The *personality* develops over the early years as a function of the interplay between the brain and the environment. By late adolescence or early adulthood, the personality stabilizes and changes very little over the remaining life span. Because of the stability of personality, when individuals do exhibit noticeable changes (e.g., becoming more outgoing, uninhibited, impulsive, socially withdrawn, apathetic), we should be concerned about frontal lobe functioning and refer for further evaluation.

The *temporal lobes* are especially important for hearing, interpreting language, learning and memory, and emotional responses. *Receptive aphasia* (inability to interpret spoken language) may result from damage to *Wernicke's area*, the functional part of the temporal cortex involved in the interpretation of language. Auditory hallucinations involve the temporal cortex, along with other structures of the brain. Located deep within the temporal cortices are important structures concerned with learning and memory. The *hippocampus* is responsible for consolidating long-term explicit memories for facts and events. *Amnesia*, defined as a severe loss of memory or learning, is reflective of injury to the hippocampus. Chronically elevated levels of cortisol, as seen in many individuals with depressive and anxiety disorders, appears to damage the hippocampus, and may be responsible for complaints related to learning and memory. Fortunately, the hippocampus is an area of the brain capable of generating new neurons, so recovery may be possible. The *amygdala* is a small structure located within the anterior medial portion of each temporal lobe that is important for detecting danger, recognizing emotions—especially negative ones—and recalling the emotional aspects of life events.

Box 6–1. Disturbances of Higher Level Cognitive Functioning

Aphasia: Disruption of language function
Apraxia: Disturbance in the organization of voluntary action (e.g., putting on one's clothes)
Agnosia: Disorganization of perception and recognition
Amnesia: Dysfunction of memory processes
Dementia: Deterioration in intellectual and cognitive functions

Functions of the *parietal lobes* include the somatosensory modalities of light touch, pressure, pain, temperature, vibration, and proprioception (position sense). The posterior portion of the parietal cortex helps us perceive and interpret spatial relationships, form an accurate body image, and learn tasks involving coordination of the body in space. When these areas become damaged, individuals may develop sensory *agnosias*, defined as the impaired ability to interpret sensory information (e.g., identifying a key in one's pocket by touch). Other examples of parietal dysfunction include graphomotor problems (e.g., drawing a clock or copying a figure) and spatial neglect (e.g., following a cerebrovascular accident). The *occipital lobes* are primarily responsible for vision. A visual agnosia is the inability to recognize objects by using vision. Visual hallucinations involve the visual cortex along with other brain structures.

Deep within the cerebrum are other important structures. The *basal ganglia* are very important nuclei for initiation of voluntary movement. The basal ganglia are outside of the descending corticospinal ("pyramidal") motor tracts and are thus considered *extrapyramidal*. When we talk about *extrapyramidal symptoms* (EPS) involving unusual movements such as *bradykinesia* (slow movement) or *hyperkinesias* (fast movement such as ticks or tremors), we are referring to symptoms that reflect dysfunction of the basal ganglia. Parkinson's disease is caused by destruction of dopaminergic neurons that project into the basal ganglia, resulting in impaired motor functioning. "Parkinsonism" is due to blockade of the same dopaminergic neurons by antipsychotics.

The *thalamus* is a relay station between the spinal cord and cortex. It transmits incoming sensory information to the relevant cortical areas. Similarly, it transmits descending motor information from the cortex to other areas of the brain and spinal cord. Together with the reticular activating system (RAS) in the brain stem, the thalamus helps modulate arousal levels. The *hypothalamus* serves as a master regulatory center in the brain, regulating food and fluid intake, temperature, and the pituitary gland via the HPA axis.

The functions of the *cerebellum* include movement, balance, and posture. The cerebellum functions to maintain equilibrium and work together with the motor cortex and basal ganglia to control movement. The cerebellum specializes in calculating the sequence of muscle contractions necessary to achieve goals in voluntary movement. When the cerebellum is dysfunctional, we may see uncoordinated and inaccurate movements such as a wide based gait (*ataxia*), difficulties touching the finger to nose, and difficulties maintaining balance (Romberg test).

The *brain stem* includes the midbrain, pons, and medulla. Neurotransmitter-producing cell bodies are clustered in the brainstem with projections that travel to diffuse areas of the brain. Brain stem cells that produce several of the neurotransmitters associated with psychiatric symptoms, disorders, and treatments include the *substantia nigra* (dopamine), *locus coeruleus* (norepinephrine), and *raphe nuclei* (serotonin). These neurotransmitter pathways are essential for modulating motor control, memory, mood, motivation, and metabolic state. The brain stem is also a major conduit for neuronal pathways that travel between the brain and periphery. The pons relays information between the cerebrum and the cerebellum. The medulla is the site of decussation (crossing over) of the descending pyramidal tracts. A brain injury below the level of decussation will have noticeable effects on the same side of the injury. A brain injury above the level of decussation will result in peripheral impairments on the opposite side of the body.

The *limbic system* is a group of brain structures important in the regulation of emotion and memory. The hippocampus and amygdala assure that we can recall the events of our lives along with their emotional valence. The olfactory system plays a very primitive role in triggering memories. In humans and primates, the frontal lobes participate in planning and decision-making parts. Disorders of emotion and memory involve the limbic structures and their connections.

Stress and the brain. The detection of threat by the amygdala triggers the hypothalamus to set off the stress response. The stress response involves two different major pathways: the ANS and the HPA axis. Activation of the ANS leads to the release of peripheral epinephrine (also called adrenalin) from the adrenal medulla. Epinephrine increases the heart rate and blood pressure and prepares us to escape the perceived danger. This response, often called the *fight or flight* response, is frequently accompanied by *fright* or anxiety. Hans Selye, in his theory of the *general adaptation syndrome* (Selye, 1956), referred to this stage as the *alarm* reaction. If the stressor can be resolved, the alarm response subsides. If not resolved, the *resistance* stage is the body's continuing attempts to adapt. If adaptation fails, the eventual outcome is the stage of *exhaustion* and illness.

The second stress pathway is the HPA axis (Figure 6–1). The hypothalamus releases corticotrophin-releasing hormone (CRH), which triggers the pituitary gland to produce adrenocorticotropic hormone (ACTH). ACTH stimulates the adrenal glands to release cortisol. Cortisol works more slowly to increase the utilization of glucose and decrease inflammation— both important for dealing with acute stressors. If all goes well, active coping leads to a resolution of the stressor. The adaptive responses to stress have been referred to by McEwen (2008) as "allostasis." If the stressor is not resolved, wear and tear on the body increases (allostatic load) with continued cortisol secretion and risk for hyperglycemia, hyperinsulinemia, hypertension, increased cholesterol, and eventually arteriosclerosis. The hippocampus, particularly sensitive to cortisol, may experience atrophy with resultant problems with memory. In summary, although the stress response is protective and adaptive, chronic activation causes increasing wear and tear on the body and eventual pathophysiology.

Figure 6–1. HPA Axis

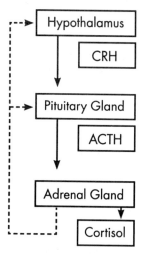

Neurons, Neurotransmitters, and Neurotransmitter Pathways

The brain tissue consists of two distinct types of cells: glia and neurons. The *glia* are the supporting structures of the brain, outnumbering neurons in a 10:1 ratio. In addition to providing support, they are important in guiding the migration of neurons during development and controlling the extracellular concentrations of potassium (K^+) and other ions. Some glia form the protective sheaths around the axons of neurons. This protective coating, *myelin*, is what we refer to as white matter, whereas the uncoated neuronal cell bodies appear more gray and are referred to as gray matter.

Though less numerous, *neurons* are considered to be the more important "microprocessors" of the brain. They are responsible for the majority of the communication among structures of the brain and among the brain and other body parts. Though the exact number is unknown, there are estimated to be some 100 billion neurons in the brain. Each neuron receives input from tens of thousands of different neurons. The complexity is nearly unfathomable.

Neurons look and act differently than other cells. In common with most other cells in the body, they have nuclei that contain DNA. All cell bodies also contain liquid cytoplasm that surrounds the nuclei, and organelles that function to produce necessary proteins. Two regions of the neuron distinguish it from other common cells. The *dendrites*, having the appearance of branches, receive information from other cells. The *axons*, generally covered with myelin, send information to other cells. Myelin insulates the axons and allows the electrical signals (axon potentials) to travel quickly down the axon, regenerating at small breaks (nodes of Ranvier) in the myelin, until they reach the terminal.

Neurotransmitters. Once the electrical action potential reaches the neuron terminal, the release of neurotransmitter is triggered. The chemical neurotransmitter diffuses across the small space between the neurons (called the *synapse*) and activates the *receptors* of the post-synaptic cell. Each neurotransmitter has a specific mechanism for inactivation once it has activated the receptor and been released back into the synapse; it either diffuses out of the synapse, gets pumped back into the terminal for recycling, or gets broken down by enzymes such as monoamine oxidase (MAO).

Although more than 40 different neurotransmitters have been found to have CNS functions, the ones that we are most familiar with in psychiatric practice are the monoamines (Table 6–2). These include acetylcholine (ACh), dopamine (DA), norepinephrine (NE), epinephrine (E), and serotonin (5-HT). Even smaller amino acids that act as CNS neurotransmitters include glutamate, and gamma-aminobutyric acid (GABA). The monoamines and amino acid neurotransmitters can be produced right in the terminals where they will be used. Larger neuroactive peptides (large protein neurotransmitters such as beta-endorphin) are only produced in the cytoplasm of the nucleus and must be transported to the terminals.

Table 6-2. Monoamine and Amino Acid Neurotransmitters and Their Functions

Neurotransmitter	Partial List of Known Functions
Dopamine	Attention and executive functioning, motivated behaviors (reward- and pleasure-seeking), addictions, mood, movement, psychosis
Norepinephrine	Arousal, concentration, learning and memory, mood, stress response
Epinephrine (adrenaline)	Peripheral activation and arousal, fight or flight response

Continued

Table 6–2. Monoamine and Amino Acid Neurotransmitters and Their Functions (cont.)

Neurotransmitter	Partial List of Known Functions
Serotonin	Mood, anxiety, appetite, eating behavior, sleep
Acetylcholine	Arousal, cognition, memory, contraction of skeletal muscle
Glutamate	Excitation
GABA	Inhibition

PATHOPHYSIOLOGY OF MENTAL DISORDERS

Pathophysiology is concerned with alterations in function that accompany a particular syndrome or disease. The pathophysiology of each of the mental disorders is a function of alterations in brain function. The average age of onset of all of the adult psychiatric disorders is in early adulthood.

The Stress-Diathesis Theory of Mental Disorders

No mental disorder can be explained by a single gene. The heritability of mental disorders ranges from as low as 29% for depression to as high as 89% for bipolar disorder (Box 6–2). Rather, each mental disorder is probably associated with a number of vulnerability genes. Whether the genes will actually be expressed, resulting in symptoms of mental illness, may depend upon environmental factors. The stress-diathesis theory of mental disorders describes contributions of genetics (diathesis) and environment (stress). The term, diathesis, describes the tendency, vulnerability, or predisposition toward psychiatric symptoms based upon genetics. Stress refers to the environmental contributions. Early life stressors such as childhood trauma or neglect, significant loss, and possibly viruses or toxins, are important environmental contributors to mental disorders. Parental behaviors that might contribute to the risk for mental disorders in their offspring include starvation, poor nutrition, lack of vitamin D exposure, and substance abuse. For individuals who have a strong genetic disposition to develop a mental condition, it may not take much of a stressor to trigger the expression of the condition. Schizophrenia and bipolar disorder are the most heritable of the mental disorders. For individuals who are less vulnerable to mental disorders, it may take a larger number or greater intensity of stressors to trigger the onset. Some disorders such as posttraumatic stress disorder (PTSD) and phobias may be triggered by exposure to extreme stress in individuals with otherwise very little vulnerability.

Box 6-2. Heritability of Mental Disorders

Highest heritability
Schizophrenia (82%–84%) (Kendler, 2001)
Bipolar disorder (85%–89%) (McGuffin, Rijsdijk, Andrew, Sham, Katz, & Cardno, 2003)

Medium heritability
Alcoholism (52%–58%) (Kendler, 2001)

Lowest heritability
Anxiety disorders (37%–43%) (Kendler, 2001)
Major depression (29%–42%) (Kendler, Gatz, Gardner, & Pedersen, 2006)

Schizophrenia

The average age of onset for schizophrenia is 18–25 for males and 25–35 for females (American Psychological Association, 2000). Although rare, children and middle-aged adults also can develop the disorder. The date of onset is defined by the 6-month period of positive symptoms; however, the prodrome period leading up to the first acute episode may last days to years. Family members often can look back after the diagnosis of schizophrenia and identify a period of altered behavior leading up to the first major episode of psychosis. During this time, a teenager may withdraw from family or friends, use drugs, and exhibit changes in motivation and school performance. Subtle delays in language and motor skills may even have been present early in life. Following an acute episode of psychosis, recovery to previous levels of functioning may be incomplete, often characterized by the persistence of negative symptoms. The three major symptom categories of schizophrenia that reflect brain abnormalities are the positive symptoms (hallucinations, delusions, abnormal speech, abnormal behavior), negative symptoms (amotivation, apathy, anhedonia), and cognitive dysfunction (diminished executive functioning and working memory).

Neurodevelopmental abnormalities. Researchers have determined that very subtle early symptoms of schizophrenia may have been present from early childhood, including delayed language development and asymmetrical use of major muscles of the body. These early findings have led researchers to the hypothesis that schizophrenia is a neurodevelopmental condition. In other words, the brains of individuals who develop schizophrenia may not develop normally. It has been hypothesized that the early migration of neurons in brain development may be faulty, resulting in abnormal connections. Support for the neurodevelopmental theory comes from the observation that during the late teens, when most individuals develop full access to the frontal executive functions of the brain, the individual with schizophrenia starts to demonstrate disordered thinking.

Neurodegenerative abnormalities. In addition, the process of pruning away unnecessary connections in the brain may go awry, resulting in too much destruction of neurons and their connections. A process called *"excitotoxicity"* (Stahl, 2008) has been used to describe the potential self-destruction of neurons resulting from too much glutamate and excitatory neuronal activity. Support for a neurodegenerative mechanism in schizophrenia comes from monozygotic twin studies showing that affected twins tend to have enlarged ventricles of the brain in comparison to their healthy twin siblings. Ventricular enlargement is due to atrophy of the brain tissues creating more space for fluid in the ventricles.

Neurotransmitter abnormalities. The pathophysiology of schizophrenia is also characterized by abnormal neurotransmission. Abnormally elevated levels of dopamine in the limbic system are thought to be responsible for positive symptoms. Because dopamine is essential for learning, memory, and motivation, the negative symptoms and cognitive impairment may reflect lower than normal levels of dopamine in the prefrontal cortex. Although dopamine is the neurotransmitter most associated with schizophrenia, researchers are learning that other neurotransmitters, such as glutamate, also may have important roles.

Mood Disorders

Disorders of mood can include depression or bipolar disorder, or the less acute but long-lasting dysthymic and cyclothymic variations. The distinction between unipolar depression and bipolar depression is important because the two disorders require different treatments. Bipolar depression is more likely to have a heritable (genetic) component than unipolar depression, and a person with bipolar disorder is more likely to have had previous symptoms, treatments, or hospitalizations. Depression can occur at any age, including the first and last years of life. Although the average age for diagnosing bipolar disorder is in the late 20s or early 30s, many of the symptoms, including impulsivity and difficulty controlling emotions, can be present as early as age 5 or 6. These early symptoms of bipolar disorder are often misdiagnosed as attention deficit-hyperactivity disorder (ADHD). Mood disorders can be triggered by upsetting life events, life transitions, physical transitions or illness, and by chronic stress.

Depression: Monoamine dysregulation. Monoamines are the neurotransmitters that include serotonin (5HT), norepinephrine (NE), and dopamine (D). The hypothesis that depression is caused by a reduction or deficit in one or more of the monoamines forms the basis for treating with the traditional antidepressants. The actual mechanism of depression is probably more complicated, involving the monoamine receptors and other cellular events, including the regulation of gene expression (Stahl, 2008).

Depression: Dysregulation of the HPA axis. A second hypothesis about the pathophysiology of depression involves the stress response systems, in particular the hypothalamus-pituitary-adrenal (HPA) axis. The HPA axis appears to be the main site where genetic and environmental influences converge to cause mood disorders. Early life stressors, such as the loss of a parent, trauma, or neglect, have been shown to produce lasting effects on the HPA axis, leading to chronic difficulty managing stress, and chronically elevated levels of cortisol. The support for this hypothesis of depression is that individuals with major depressive disorder often present with hypercortisolemia, resistance of cortisol to suppression by dexamethasone, blunted ACTH responses to corticotrophin-releasing hormone (CRH) challenge, and elevated CRH concentrations in the cerebrospinal fluid (CSF).

Bipolar disorder: Monoamine dysregulation. Bipolar manic episodes may involve the same neurotransmitter systems as depression, with problems related to over-activity rather than under-activity. Elevated levels of 5HT, NE, and D in areas of the brain regulating mood and behavior could explain symptoms such as irritable or expansive mood, pressured speech, flight of ideas, decreased sleep, and increased goal-directed activity. Sensitivity and kindling are two terms that have been used to describe neuronal activity in bipolar disorder. Early in the course of the illness, mood episodes may be triggered by significant stressors. Over time, the brain appears to become sensitized to stress and much less stress is necessary to trigger an episode. The neurons respond to slight provocations like kindling wood for fire: a small puff of wind and the kindling catches on fire immediately.

Anxiety

Anxiety can be a normal emotion in threatening circumstances. It is the emotional component of the "fight or flight" stress response and has important survival functions. Anxiety can also be part of a syndrome or symptom complex associated with certain medical or substance-related conditions. Examples include hyperthyroidism, ADHD, and alcohol or benzodiazepine withdrawal. Finally, anxiety can be the primary component of a disorder. The anxiety disorders are characterized by fear and worry.

Anxiety is common at all ages. Children can develop all of the anxiety disorders experienced by adults, in addition to separation anxiety disorder. Separation anxiety is a normal stage of development around 6–18 months. However, separation anxiety becomes a disorder when school-aged children continue to express fear of separation along with significant functional impairment. Although anxiety has a heritable component, anxiety disorders such as PTSD and phobias occur following a threatening event.

Dysfunctional brain circuits related to threat perception. The neurobiology of fear is thought to involve brain circuits that are regulated by the amygdala, the small brain structure that is responsible for detecting threat and initiating the stress response. Worry may involve a different brain circuit that passes through the basal ganglia. The connection with the basal ganglia is especially important in obsessive-compulsive disorder (OCD), where we see overlap with other disorders that are linked to basal ganglia dysfunction, such as ADHD and tics.

Chronic stress response. Anxiety disorders and depression often share symptoms that are associated with a chronic stress response. Symptoms associated with chronic stress include tension headaches, migraine headaches, and musculoskeletal pain. In addition, a chronic response to stress via the HPA axis (Figure 6–1), with increased circulating levels of cortisol, has been linked to increased abdominal fat; impaired immune function; disrupted glucose metabolism; cardiovascular symptoms (e.g., hypertension); gastric ulcers; and hippocampal atrophy with learning and memory impairments.

Neurotransmitter dysregulation. We know that the brain's GABA receptors can be modulated by depressants such as alcohol and benzodiazepines. When people drink alcohol or take benzodiazepines, anxiety levels tend to subside. During withdrawal from those same substances, anxiety increases. These findings support the hypothesis that the neurotransmitter GABA and its receptors are important in the symptoms of anxiety. Too little GABA is associated with symptoms of anxiety. On the other hand, too much arousal from NE or glutamate may also lead to symptoms of anxiety.

Obesity and Eating Disorders

Obesity is associated with many health risks, including type 2 diabetes, heart disease, stroke, hypertension, osteoarthritis, sleep apnea, and some forms of cancer. Poor diet and sedentary lifestyle contribute to obesity; however, the chief contributor is heredity. The heritability of obesity is equivalent to that of height (Bear, Connors, & Paradiso, 2006), and as with all of the mental disorders, more than one gene is involved. Obesity can result from a variety of disorders that cause hormonal imbalance, including hypothyroidism, hypercortisolism, primary hyperinsulinism, pseudohypoparathyroidism, and acquired hypothalamic problems (e.g., tumors, infections, traumatic syndromes).

Recently, concern has been voiced regarding the risk of metabolic syndrome in individuals who are taking atypical antipsychotics. *Metabolic syndrome* includes the following symptoms: abdominal obesity, dyslipidemia, raised blood pressure, insulin resistance with or without glucose intolerance, proinflammatory state, and prothrombotic state. Individuals with metabolic syndrome are at risk for premature coronary heart disease.

Because many of the psychotropic medications can cause weight gain and increase the risk for metabolic syndrome, it is especially important that we monitor weight and body mass index (BMI) before and during treatment. BMI can be calculated based on weight and height, and BMI charts are readily available for both adults and children on websites such as the Centers for Disease Control and Prevention (http://www.cdc.gov/nccdphp/dnpa/healthyweight/assessing/bmi/index.htm) or the National Heart Lung and Blood Institute (http://www.nhlbisupport.com/bmi/). The normal range of BMI for adults is between 18.5 and 24.9, with 25 to 29.9 indicating overweight and anything over 30 indicating obesity.

Eating disorders. Anorexia and bulimia are eating disorders found primarily in highly developed cultures such as in the United States, especially those with a focus on youth and beauty. They are serious conditions that can be fatal if untreated. Both involve cognitive distortions around body shape and weight. Anorexia is characterized by refusal to maintain body weight at or above 85% of the expected based on age and height. Multiple physiological factors are involved in the complex regulation of eating. The self-induced state of starvation seen in anorexia has serious physical consequences including cardiac arrhythmias, bradycardia or tachycardia, hypotension, hypothermia, skin dryness with possible lanugo (a soft, fine, downy hair on the arms and other body parts that is normal in infancy), edema, and amenorrhea. Basically, all organ systems are affected by starvation. Hospitalization is indicated for patients who are 20% or more below the expected weight for their height.

Bulimia is characterized by recurrent episodes of binge eating followed by inappropriate compensatory mechanisms. Vomiting or laxative abuse can lead to metabolic disturbances and electrolyte abnormalities (e.g., hypokalemia, hypochloremic alkalosis, hypomagnesemia). Recurrent self-induced vomiting can result in the loss of dental enamel, scars on the hand, and esophageal tears.

Addictions

Genetic factors and environmentally induced alterations in brain neurochemistry appear to influence vulnerability for addiction. Addictions are a chronic, relapsing disease of the brain characterized by compulsive drug-seeking and use (Volkow, 2008). All drugs of abuse are thought to increase brain dopamine in the pathways that drive motivation and reward. Chronic use of alcohol or other drugs may produce alterations in brain neurochemistry that help to maintain addictive behaviors. Higher rates of substance abuse are found in impulsive groups: violent offenders, conduct disorder, intermittent explosive disorder. Stress increases alcohol and drug use, and is associated with higher rates of relapse. Substance use disorders are frequently comorbid with other mental disorders. For further information about the effects of specific substances on brain neurophysiology, visit the website of the National Institute on Drug Abuse: http://www.nida.nih.gov.

Attention Deficit-Hyperactivity Disorder (ADHD)

Attention deficit-hyperactivity disorder (ADHD) is characterized by inattentiveness, impulsiveness, and hyperactivity. By definition, the symptoms must be present before age 7, but the diagnosis can be made at any age. Possible risk factors for the development of ADHD include genetics, perinatal complications, neurologic illness, diet, allergy, and environmental toxins. The neurobiology of ADHD is complex. ADHD is highly comorbid with anxiety, depression, and other mental disorders. The overlap of ADHD with obsessive compulsive behaviors and motor tics suggests that the basal ganglia and the motor pathway that produces dopamine and travels to the basal ganglia (the nigrostriatal pathway) are involved. In addition, executive functioning problems (impulsivity, impaired attentional and organizational skills) suggest frontal lobe abnormalities. The neurotransmitters that have been associated with the attentional and hyperactivity deficits are dopamine and norepinephrine, and with impulsivity, serotonin.

Dementia

There are many different types of dementia, including Alzheimer's, Lewy body, frontotemporal, and HIV. The most common cause of dementia is Alzheimer's disease (AD). Nearly 10% of individuals over the age of 65 and 25% to 40% of individuals over the age of 85 have AD (Breitner et al., 1999). Early changes in Alzheimer's disease and other dementias appear to be related to a decrease in the brain's levels of acetylcholine (ACh), a neurotransmitter essential to learning and memory. Support for this assumption comes from the observation that boosting cholinergic functioning with cholinesterase inhibitors (therefore reducing the metabolism and increasing the availability) enhances memory function in early dementia. As Alzheimer's dementia progresses, deposits of a protein called amyloid, and bundles of tangled proteins called neurofibrillary tangles, begin to interfere with the functioning of neuronal cells. The process of excitotoxicity related to glutamate overactivity is also thought to be responsible for some of the neurodegeneration and atrophy of the brain seen on MRI scans.

There are many differences between the pathophysiologies of the different dementias. *Lewy body dementia* is more common in individuals with Parkinson's disease and is characterized by the deposition of Lewy bodies (a protein) in the neurons. Individuals with Lewy body dementia may have visual hallucinations, a characteristic that distinguishes them from other dementias. *Frontotemporal (Pick's)* dementia is characterized by atrophy in the frontal and temporal brain regions due to neuronal loss, gliosis, and Pick's bodies (masses of cytoskeletal elements). A distinguishing characteristic of *vascular dementia* is that cognitive functioning may decline in a stair-step (rather than progressive) fashion following cerebrovascular accidents.

In HIV-infected individuals, a dementia can result from the direct effects of HIV infection in the brain, opportunistic infections, or the toxic effects of drug treatments. The HIV virus may gain entrance to the CNS by infecting the macrophages and monocytes that cross the blood–brain barrier. Symptoms of the resulting AIDS dementia complex can be confused with clinical depression due to the presentation of apathy and cognitive and motor problems.

Delirium

Delirium is a serious medical condition that can be caused by any number of disturbances (see the "I Watch Death" mnemonic in Box 6–3). Unlike dementia, which is generally a slowly progressing condition, delirium can come on rapidly and is characterized by a clouding of consciousness with disorientation. Whereas someone with dementia may remain relatively oriented until the later stages of the illness, individuals with delirium may shift between periods of orientation and disorientation.

Box 6-3. I WATCH DEATH: A Mnemonic

- Infection
- Withdrawal
- Acute metabolic disturbance
- Trauma
- CNS pathology
- Hypoxia
- Deficiencies
- Endocrinopathies
- Acute vascular
- Toxins
- Heavy metals

Sundowning is the term used for the disorientation that individuals with dementia may experience when familiar environmental cues diminish with nighttime. If delirium is suspected, it is important to alert the medical team so a complete physical assessment can be completed. Often, in older persons, an infection such as pneumonia or a urinary tract infection is found to be the culprit.

Comorbidities

Mental disorders are frequently comorbid with each other. Examples include depression and anxiety (Stahl, 2008); eating disorders and depression (Stahl, 2008); and dementia and depression, anxiety, or psychosis (Kverno, Rabins, Blass, Hicks, & Black, 2008). According to the National Institute of Drug Abuse (NIDA, 2007), patients with mood or anxiety disorders are about twice as likely to also suffer from a drug disorder. The highest comorbidity appears to be with mania, with nearly 40% of affected individuals having a lifetime prevalence of a drug disorder (NIDA, 2007). Pediatric diagnoses can be atypical, constantly changing, and unusually comorbid with other psychiatric disorders. ADHD, for example, is frequently comorbid with anxiety, depression, conduct disorder, oppositional behavior, substance abuse, and tics (Stahl, 2008).

Human Sexuality, Sexual Dysfunction, and Risks

The three phases of the sexual response cycle—libido, arousal, and orgasm—all have distinct and relatively non-overlapping neurotransmitter functions (Stahl, 2008). Each stage of the cycle can be affected by mental disorders or their treatments. Depression and anxiety are commonly associated with sexual dysfunction. Manic episodes may result in increased libido and sexual behavior. Of the neurotransmitter systems that we have discussed in relation to the mental disorders, dopamine and the brain reward pathways are thought to play a role in increasing libido or sexual desire. Serotonin has a negative influence, and norepinephrine a positive influence, on sexual arousal and orgasm. When we consider that most of the psychotropic drugs affect these three neurotransmitter systems, it is not surprising that sexual dysfunction is often an unwanted side effect of treatment.

Sexually transmitted diseases include syphilis, gonorrhea, chlamydia, trichomoniasis, human papillomavirus (HPV), herpes simplex virus, and HIV. HPV causes genital warts, and is associated with an increased risk for cervical cancer. A new HPV vaccine is available to girls ages 11 and older. Syphilis is caused by a spirochetal bacterium that, if not diagnosed or treated, can cause dementia via the slow, progressive infection of the brain.

Vulnerable populations at risk for HIV are individuals who have unprotected sex with multiple partners, IV drug users, gay men, hemophiliacs, and children born to HIV+ women. The routes of transmission of HIV are the blood and body fluids, usually through sexual contact, contaminated IV needles, or transfusions. Once inside the body, the HIV virus targets the CD4 receptor on the T4 lymphocytes. The virus injects its RNA into the infected lymphocyte and becomes part of cell division, eventually disabling the patient's T4 lymphocytes and impairing immune functioning. About 6 months after exposure, the individual can test positive for HIV. Therefore, those at risk need to be tested about every 6 months. The Centers for Disease Control and Prevention (CDC) recommends a diagnosis of AIDS when the T4 concentration falls to 20% of normal. The diagnosis of AIDS is also made following an opportunistic infection, sometimes up to 10 to 17 years after exposure to HIV. New antiretroviral drugs have lengthened the time from exposure to the development of AIDS and AIDS dementia.

REFERENCES

American Psychological Association. (2000). *Diagnostic and statistical manual of mental disorders* (4th ed., rev. ed.). Washington, DC: Author.

Bear, M., Connors, B., & Paradiso, M. (2006). *Neuroscience: Exploring the brain* (3rd ed.). Baltimore: Lippincott Williams & Wilkins.

Breitner, J., Wyse, B., Anthony, J., Welsh-Bohmer, K., Steffens, D., Norton, M., et al. (1999). APOE-epsilon4 count predicts age when prevalence of AD increases, then declines: The Cache County Study. *Neurology, 53*(2), 321–331.

Kendler, K. (2001). Twin studies of psychiatric illness. *Archives of General Psychiatry, 58,* 1005–1014.

Kendler, K., Gatz, M., Gardner, C., & Pedersen, N. (2006). A Swedish national twin study of lifetime major depression. *American Journal of Psychiatry, 163*(1), 109–114.

Kverno, K., & Goertz, S. (2007). Neurobiologic considerations in psychiatric care. In P. O'Brien, W. Kennedy, & K. Ballard (Eds.), *Psychiatric–mental health nursing. An introduction to theory and practice* (pp. 65–88). Sudbury, MA: Jones and Bartlett.

Kverno, K., Rabins, P., Blass, D., Hicks, K., & Black, B. (2008). Prevalence and treatment of neuropsychiatric symptoms in hospice-eligible nursing home residents with advanced dementia. *Journal of Gerontological Nursing, 34*(12), 8–15.

McEwen, B. S. (2007). Physiology and neurobiology of stress and adaptation: Central role of the brain. *Physiological Reviews, 87,* 873–904.

McGuffin, P., Rijsdijk, F., Andrew, M., Sham, P., Katz, R., & Cardno, A. (2003). The heritability of bipolar affective disorder and the genetic relationship to unipolar depression. *Archives of General Psychiatry, 60*(5), 497–502.

National Institute on Drug Abuse. (October, 2007). *Topics in brief. Comorbid drug abuse and mental illness.* Retrieved January 8, 2009, from http://www.nida.nih.gov/pdf/tib/comorbid.pdf

Selye, H. (1956). *The stress of life.* New York: McGraw-Hill.

Stahl, S. (2008). *Stahl's essential psychopharmacology: Neuroscientific basis and practical applications.* New York: Cambridge University Press.

Volkow, N. (2008). *Director's message to medical and health professionals. National Institute on Drug Abuse.* Retrieved January 8, 2009, from http://www.nida.nih.gov/about/welcome/medstaffmessage.html

Psychopharmacology

Karan Kverno, PhD, PMHNP-BC, PMHCNS-BC

Standard 5D of the American Nurses Association's (2007) *Scope and Standards of Psychiatric–Mental Health Nursing Practice* is related to psychopharmacology. The psychiatric–mental health RN is expected to: 1) apply current research findings to guide nursing actions related to pharmacology; 2) assess patients' responses to biological interventions based on current knowledge of pharmacological agents' intended actions, interactive effects, potential untoward effects, and therapeutic doses; 3) provide health teaching for medication management; 4) provide health teaching about mechanism of action, intended effects, potential adverse effects, ways to cope with transitional side effects, and other treatment options; 5) direct interventions toward alleviating untoward effects of biological interventions; and 6) communicate observations about patients' responses to biological interventions to other health clinicians. Your basic knowledge of the biological basis of psychiatric illness from Chapter 6 will be essential for understanding the therapeutic and adverse effects of psychopharmacology.

Safe Medication Management

As part of the Quality Chasm Series, the Institute of Medicine published *To Err Is Human* (2000), a summary of research findings on the unacceptable level of medication errors in hospitals. This was followed in 2007 by *Preventing Medication Errors*. These two important reports, in combination with the Joint Commission's 2009 National Patient Safety Goals, provide evidence-based strategies for preventing medication errors. The recommendations include: 1) patient-centered care with improved provider–patient communication about medication benefits and risks; 2) maintaining a complete medication list with important information concerning medication name, dose, route, frequency, duration, and start date; 3) reviewing the patient's medication list routinely and during care transitions; 4) electronic prescribing and monitoring; and 5) adopting an organizational culture of safety. Organizations are expected to identify and take actions to prevent errors from medications that look or sound alike, avoid the use of confusing abbreviations and symbols, and label all medications and containers. The official "Do Not Use" list for confusing abbreviations can be found on the Joint Commission's website.

PHARMACOKINETICS AND PHARMACODYNAMICS

Pharmacokinetics

Pharmacokinetics refers to what the body does to a drug: absorption, distribution, metabolism, and excretion. For most psychiatric drugs, the principle route of administration is oral. Oral drugs are absorbed through the small bowel, passing into the portal circulation and liver. Most of the psychotropic drugs are partially metabolized by the cytochrome P450 enzymes as the drugs pass through the liver. This process is called "first-pass metabolism" and is avoided by drugs that are given IV or IM. After the first pass through the liver, the drugs enter systemic circulation, where they are distributed to organs in direct proportion to their fat and protein content. Most psychotropic drugs are highly lipophilic and highly protein-bound. The unbound (free) concentration of the drug then readily passes the blood-brain barrier. These drugs also have rapid and extensive distribution in other tissue compartments.

Many factors affect pharmacokinetics, including alterations in hepatic cytochrome P450 enzyme concentrations, kidney functioning, the amount of bound protein in the circulation, the half-life of the drug, and the time to onset of action.

- Hepatic cytochrome P450 enzyme interactions can induce or inhibit the metabolism of certain drugs, changing the desired concentration levels. For example, nicotine is an inducer of P450 enzymes, so heavy smokers may require a lower dose of a drug after they quit smoking. Hepatic disease will affect liver enzyme activity and first-pass metabolism. For drugs that have high first-pass effects, hepatic disease can result in elevated or toxic plasma drug levels.
- Some drugs rely more on excretion by the kidneys than metabolism by the liver. Renal disease or drugs that reduce renal clearance (e.g., NSAIDs) may increase serum concentration of these drugs (e.g., lithium).
- The amount of free-circulating drug determines the effect of the drug, not the drug that is bound to proteins in the bloodstream. If a highly protein-bound drug is displaced off its protein by another, more strongly protein-bound drug, it can result in increased circulating levels of the first drug. Any condition that shifts the ratio of bound to free drug can change the concentration of drug (e.g., malnutrition, wasting, aging).

- *Half-life* is the time needed to clear 50% of a drug from the plasma. It also determines the length of time necessary to reach steady state and how frequently drugs must be taken to maintain the desired effect. Steady state is reached when the amount administered per unit time equals the amount eliminated per unit time. It takes five half-lives for concentration to build to steady state. Likewise, it takes five half-lives to wash out a drug. Half-life is a determinant of the duration of action of a drug.
- *Onset of action* is the length of time that it takes for a medicine to start to work. Drugs within a category may be chosen based upon their onset of action. For example, sedatives with rapid onset of action will be useful for individuals with sleep-onset insomnia.
- Age and gender affect how the body processes drugs.
  - *Children* often have greater hepatic capacity, more glomerular filtration, and less fatty tissue. In addition, they may be less able to store drugs in their fat, resulting in quicker elimination and shorter half-lives. These differences in children and adolescents may result in recommended dosages that approach those of adults despite smaller body size.
  - In contrast, *older adults* have less efficient livers and kidneys, resulting in slower metabolism and excretion of drugs. In addition, most of the psychotropic drugs are lipid-soluble, so due to the loss of lean body mass and increase in body fat concentration, the lipid-soluble psychotropic drugs distribute widely in fat tissue, unexpectedly prolonging drug actions.
  - Besides kidney and liver changes, *older adults* have lower levels of functioning in most organ systems compared to their younger adult counterparts. Cardiovascular disease and reduced cardiac output can affect both renal and hepatic drug clearance. Cardiovascular disease especially increases the risks of using drugs with potential cardiac effects (e.g., tricyclics). A common side effect of many of the psychotropic drugs, orthostatic hypotension, greatly increases the risk for falls in the elderly. Gastrointestinal disease and decreased gastric acid secretion may slow absorption. Brain changes and reduced acetylcholine (ACh) output increase the risk for anticholinergic toxicity. In general, the elderly are more susceptible to adverse drug effects and interactions (particularly cardiac).
  - For *women*, the periods of life associated with pregnancies and menopause carry certain pharmacological risks. Positive pregnancy tests are possible at weeks 4 to 7, but may be past the window of teratogenic risk. Most malformations occur during the embryonic period (weeks 3–8 of gestation). Overall, the recommendations to women of childbearing age are to prevent first-trimester exposure to psychotropic medications by using birth control. If pregnancy occurs and psychotropic drugs must be used during pregnancy, the antipsychotics may be safer than antidepressants, mood stabilizers, or lithium. Antidepressant prophylaxis during the third trimester may be used to prevent postpartum depression in women with history of depression. Because of lipid solubility, psychotropic drugs pass readily into breastmilk, so mothers must be advised of alternatives.

Pharmacodynamics

Pharmacodynamics refers to what the drug does to the body. The brain structures involved in pharmacodynamics include the receptors, ion channels, enzymes, and transport pumps.

Receptors. Psychotherapeutic drugs produce a wide range of adverse effects on neurotransmitter receptors. Each neurotransmitter has several receptor types, and each given receptor type may have multiple subtypes with different actions. Thus, one drug can have multiple actions in different areas of the brain and spinal cord, depending on the distribution of neurotransmitter pathways and receptors. As newer drugs are developed with greater selectivity and specificity, they have fewer unwanted (side) effects.

- Anticholinergic: Blockade of muscarinic acetylcholine receptors
- Extrapyramidal side effects (EPS): Antagonism of D2 receptors
- Sedation: Blockade of histamine receptors
- Orthostatic hypotension: Blockade of adrenergic receptors
- Sexual dysfunction, anxiety, akathisia, insomnia, GI upset, and diarrhea, due to excessive activation of serotonergic receptors

Ion channels. Channels exist for many ions, including sodium, potassium, chloride, and calcium. Drugs such as calcium channel blockers act by blocking the movement of calcium through the channel. Unlike the ions, neurotransmitters do not actually pass from one neuron into another. Instead the neurotransmitter interacts with the receptor, causing it to change configuration. The effects of this "gating" action depend upon whether the neurotransmitter has an excitatory or inhibitory action at the receptor. For example, glutamate is an excitatory neurotransmitter. One of the glutamate receptors (NMDA) gates a calcium channel. When glutamate interacts with the NMDA receptor, calcium is allowed in, depolarizing the postsynaptic cell.

Enzymes. Enzymes are proteins important for drug metabolism. Monoamine oxidase (MAO) is an enzyme that metabolizes the monoamine neurotransmitters (5HT, D, and NE). MAO is located inside the terminals of catecholamine neurons. After the neurotransmitter is released into the synaptic cleft and reacts with the receptor, it can be pumped back into the terminal where MAO can destroy it. Antidepressant drugs that block MAO (MAO inhibitors) decrease the metabolism of monoamines in the cytosol (i.e., once they have been pumped back into the terminal), and thus increase the availability of neurotransmitter for recycling and rerelease from the neuron.

Transport pumps are proteins that actively carry neurotransmitter molecules out of the synapse and back into the presynaptic neuron. When reuptake pumps are inhibited, the concentration of certain neurotransmitters or ions builds up in the synapse or extracellular space. For example, selective serotonin reuptake inhibitors (SSRIs) block re-uptake of serotonin, increasing the synaptic availability.

PRESCRIPTION DRUGS FOR MAJOR MENTAL DISORDERS

It is useful to classify the types of drugs by the categories of disorders that they treat. However, in practice, due to the overlapping pathophysiological mechanisms (Chapter 6), the drugs are often used across categories. For example, antidepressants are used to treat anxiety disorders and eating disorders, in addition to depression. The major classes of drugs (and their most common treatment category) are as follows:

- Antipsychotics/neuroleptics (psychosis)
- Antidepressants (depression)
- Antimanic/mood stabilizers (bipolar disorder)
- Anxiolytics/sedative-hypnotics (anxiety)

- Stimulants (ADHD)
- Cognitive enhancers (dementia)

Phases of Treatment: For most disorders, the phases of treatment are as follows:
- *Acute phase:* The focus is on interventions to prevent harm, control disturbed behavior, reduce positive symptoms, return the patient as quickly as possible to best level of functioning, form an alliance with patient and family to develop mutually agreeable short- and long-term treatment goals, and begin referrals to community resources. In this phase, new medications may be started or current medications adjusted, so it is very important to monitor response and educate patient and family.
- *Stabilization phase:* The focus is on interventions to minimize stress and enhance adaptation, with continued reduction in symptoms and recovery of functioning. Adjustments may be made to medications. Continue to monitor response and side effects, providing information as necessary. During this phase, the nurse can help the patient learn self-management skills.
- *Maintenance phase:* The focus is on interventions that ensure that symptom remission or control is sustained. The goal is recovery: to maintain or improve level of functioning and quality of life. The patient is asked to report increases in symptoms or relapses, and any adverse effects from medications. Monitor weight, BMI, blood glucose, and other parameters depending upon medication side effects. Assess for abnormal involuntary movements (e.g., AIM Scale), and return of mood or behavioral symptoms.

ANTIPSYCHOTICS

Conventional Antipsychotics: Dopamine Receptor Antagonists

Conventional antipsychotics were the first generation of antipsychotics, but are no longer considered first-line treatments due to their side effect profiles.

Indications: Positive symptoms, including psychosis, manic excitation, severe agitation, and tics and vocal utterances in Tourette syndrome. Additionally, in children: severely agitated, combative, or explosive behaviors.
- *The mechanism of action* is widespread antagonism of dopamine receptors, especially the D2 receptor. The intended target for blocking dopamine is in the limbic system; however, these drugs tend to block dopamine in dopamine pathways that serve other brain areas as well, resulting in Parkinsonism (basal ganglia), increased negative symptoms (prefrontal cortex), and hyperprolactinemia (pituitary gland).
- There are at least 20 different conventional antipsychotics (Box 7–1). They are all similarly effective, yet their side effect profiles differ. They also have a wide range of potency.
- High-potency conventional antipsychotics have a greater risk for extrapyramidal symptoms (EPS), but less sedation and anticholinergic side effects than atypical antipsychotics.
- High-potency antipsychotics can be used as depot (decanoate) injections. These typically only need to be given every 3 to 4 weeks. Available decanoate antipsychotics include haloperidol (Haldol), fluphenazine (Prolixin), and one of the more potent 2nd-generation antipsychotics, risperidone (Risperdal).

- *Clinical response:* Clinical effects in 30 to 60 minutes, antipsychotic action in 7–10 days, full therapeutic effect in 4 to 6 weeks. Conventional antipsychotics have long half-lives and are eliminated slowly.

Box 7–1. Conventional Antipsychotics Still in Use

Generic Name	Trade Name
chlorpromazine	Thorazine
cyamemazine	Tercian
flupentixol	Depixol
fluphenazine	Prolixin
haloperidol	Haldol
loxapine	Loxitane
mesoridazine	Serentil
molindone	Moban
perphenazine	Trilafon
pimozide	Orap
pipotiazine	Piportil
sulpiride	Dolmatil
thioridazine	Mellaril
thiothixene	Navane
trifluoperazine	Stelazine
zuclopenthixol	Clopixol

Adapted from *Stahl's essential psychopharmacology: Neuroscientific basis and practical applications* (3rd ed.), by S. Stahl, 2008, New York: Cambridge University Press.

Conventional Antipsychotics: Potential Adverse Effects and Their Treatments

- *Anticholinergic side effects and nursing interventions:* Anticholinergic medications decrease the availability of ACh and dry out mucus membranes.
  - *Constipation:* Encourage high dietary fiber and increased water intake. Give laxatives as ordered.
  - *Dry mouth:* Advise frequent sips of water. Provide sugarless hard candies, gum, mouth rinses.
  - *Nasal congestion:* Saline spray may help. Give over-the-counter nasal decongestant if appropriate.
  - *Blurred vision:* Advise patient to avoid potentially dangerous tasks. Reassure patient that normal vision typically returns in a few weeks, when tolerance to anticholinergic side effects develops. Pilocarpine eye drops can be used on a short-term basis.
  - *Urinary retention:* May require bethanechol.
- *Nursing interventions for other possible side effects:*
  - *Sedation:* Help patient get up and moving. Give drug at bedtime rather than in morning.
  - *GI discomfort:* Give drug with meals if not contraindicated.

- *Hypotension or orthostatic hypotension:* Advise to get out of bed slowly. Measure BP prior to dose.
- *Weight gain:* Teach about risks, encourage exercise and healthy diet.
- *Increased prolactin* levels leading to breast enlargement and galactorrhea: This can be especially troublesome to adolescents. Report, reassure. Patient may need to be switched to a different drug.

• *Extrapyramidal side effects (EPS) of conventional antipsychotics:* EPS (chemically induced Parkinsonism, dystonia, and akathisia) result from blockade of D2 receptors in the dopamine nigrostriatal pathway.
- *Parkinsonism:* Muscle stiffness, cogwheel rigidity, shuffling gait, stooped posture, drooling, slow resting tremor.
- *Dystonia:* Slow, sustained muscle contractions or spasms. Can result in oculogyric crisis, blepharospasm, and glossopharyngeal dystonias.
- *Akathisia:* A subjective feeling of muscular discomfort and restlessness.

• *Medication management of EPS:* Monitoring patients for the development of EPS is made easier by the use of standardized instruments, such as the Abnormal Involuntary Movement Scale (AIMS). When used regularly, the AIMS helps in detecting the onset of EPS. Once EPS are recognized, a variety of medications can be used to treat the symptoms. If the EPS can be treated successfully, there may be no need to discontinue the antipsychotic, assuming the patient is responding well otherwise. Medications used to treat EPS are as follows:
- *Anticholinergic agents:* Benztropine (Cogentin); trihexyphenidyl (Artane)
- *Antihistamines:* Diphenhydramine (Benadryl)
- *Dopamine agonists:* Amantadine (Symmetrel)
- *Alpha-adrenergic agonists:* Clonidine (Catapres); guanfacine (Tenex)
- *Beta-adrenergic antagonists:* Propranolol (Inderal)
- *Benzodiazepines:* Clonazepam (Klonopin); lorazepam (Ativan)

• *Tardive dyskinesia:* Occurs in 10% to 20% of patients who are treated for more than 1 year and rarely occurs until after 6 months of treatment. Consists of abnormal, involuntary movements; perioral are the most common. Regular monitoring with the AIMS or similar standardized measures will aid in detecting symptoms early so antipsychotic dosage can be decreased or the patient can be switched to a different medication, generally an atypical antipsychotic.

• *Neuroleptic malignant syndrome (NMS):* A rare, life-threatening complication that can occur any time during treatment. Motor and behavioral symptoms include muscular rigidity and dystonia, akinesia, mutism, obtundation, and agitation. Autonomic symptoms include hyperpyrexia, sweating, and increased pulse and blood pressure. If a patient taking an antipsychotic medication presents with these symptoms, the treatment includes immediate discontinuation of dopamine receptor antagonist drugs; medical support to cool the patient; monitoring of vital signs, electrolytes, fluid balance, and renal output; and symptomatic treatment of fevers.

- *Anticholinergic toxicity:* Anticholinergic symptoms are common with many of the antipsychotics, but if they increase to the point of toxicity, they can be life-threatening. A useful mnemonic for remembering the symptoms is "Dry as a bone, red as a beet, hot as a hare, blind as a bat, and mad as a hatter." People may become agitated. Because ACh is so important to cognitive functioning, the lack of it creates severe cognitive symptoms including possible disorientation to time, person, and place, as well as hallucinations. Seizures, stupor, and coma may ensue. The elderly are especially vulnerable. Regular monitoring of anticholinergic symptoms will help prevent toxicity. If symptoms of toxicity do arise, discontinue the causative agents, provide close medical supervision, and give medication (physostigmine) to reverse symptoms.

Atypical Antipsychotics: Serotonin-Dopamine Antagonists (SDAs)

The atypical antipsychotics have two major "atypical" features compared to the conventional antipsychotics: they have a lower risk for EPS and they are better for treating the negative symptoms of schizophrenia. There are five different atypical antipsychotics, all similarly effective yet their side effect profiles differ. The atypical antipsychotics have become the first-line treatments for psychotic disorders. They are also approved as mood stabilizers for the treatment of bipolar mania and depression. For children, atypical antipsychotics are faster and more robust than lithium and anticonvulsants and may be used as first-line treatments for mania.

- *Indications:*
  - *Positive symptoms:* Psychosis, manic excitation, severe agitation, severe behavioral disturbances in children and in individuals with dementia (see black box warning) or impulse control problems.
  - *Mood stabilization:* Bipolar maintenance, bipolar depression, or unresponsive unipolar depression in combination with an antidepressant
- *Mechanism of action:* Dopamine antagonism is not as robust at the D2 receptor, and therefore, has a much lower risk for EPS, negative symptoms, and hyperprolactinemia than the typical antipsychotics. Because of the inhibitory action of serotonin on dopamine-producing cells, the additional serotonin receptor antagonism of the atypical antipsychotics may actually improve dopaminergic functioning in the prefrontal regions of the brain, thus, improving negative symptoms.
- Atypical antipsychotics include clozapine (Clozaril), risperidone (Risperdal), olanzapine (Zyprexa), quetiapine (Seroquel), and ziprasidone (Geodon). Aripiprazole (Abilify) also falls into the atypical category, although the mechanism of action is a bit different (D2 receptor partial agonist). Examples of new atypical antipsychotics include paliperidone (an active metabolite of risperidone, brand name Invega), loxapine (Loxapac or Loxitane), sertindole (Serdolect), and amisulpride (Solian).

Atypical Antipsychotic (SDAs): Adverse Effects and Treatments

- *Common side effects:* Hypersomnia/sedation. Occasional EPS but much less common than with the conventional antipsychotics.

- *Metabolic syndrome:*
  - The risk for cardiometabolic changes includes increased appetite, increased weight gain, increased triglycerides, insulin resistance, hyperinsulinemia, prediabetes, diabetes, cardiovascular events, and shortened lifespan. Cardiometabolic risk is highest for clozapine and olanzapine and lowest for ziprasidone and aripiprazole.
  - Baseline: Before beginning an atypical antipsychotic, measure weight, waist circumference, blood pressure, fasting plasma glucose, and fasting lipid profile. Ask about personal and family history of obesity, dyslipidemia, hypertension, and cardiovascular disease.
  - During treatment: Monitor weight and BMI, fasting glucose, and blood pressure.
  - Promote exercise programs and dietary management.
  - Consider switching to another atypical antipsychotic for patients who become overweight, obese, prediabetic, diabetic, hypertensive, or dyslipidemic while receiving an atypical antipsychotic.
- *Black box warning:* Elderly patients with dementia-related psychosis treated with atypical antipsychotic drugs are at increased risk of death compared to placebo.
- *Drug-specific side/adverse effects:*
  - *Clozapine (Clozaril, Leponex)* was the first atypical antipsychotic on the market. It works well, but has a number of potentially serious side effects.
    - Due to side effects, it is not a first-line treatment choice. May reduce positive symptoms in patients who do not respond to other antipsychotics. May reduce tardive dyskinesia.
    - Notable side effects: Increased risk for metabolic syndrome, increased salivation, and sweating.
    - Risk for life-threatening adverse reactions:
      - Agranulocytosis (includes flu-like symptoms, sore throat, or signs of infection). Suspend treatment if white blood cell count falls below 2,000/mm3
      - Seizures: Risk increases with dose
    - *Interventions/nursing implications:* Because of the risk of agranulocytosis, monitor WBC count weekly; reduce to biweekly monitoring after 6 months. Monitor weight, blood pressure, fasting plasma glucose and lipids, ECG. The usual dosage range: 300–450 mg/day (may go as high as 900mg).
  - *Risperidone (Risperdal):* Comes in a long-acting IM decanoate form under the name Consta, which only needs to be given once every 2 weeks. Risk for EPS if dose above 6 mg/day.
  - *Quetiapine (Seroquel):* The most sedating. May be helpful to psychotic patients with sleep disorder.
  - *Ziprasidone (Geodon):* May have activating effects at low doses. Risk of QTc prolongation; monitor ECG.
  - *Aripiprazole (Abilify):* Is also approved for adjunctive therapy to antidepressants for major depressive disorder in adults.
- *Clinical Response:* Psychotic symptoms can improve within 1 week, but it may take several weeks for full effect on behavior. Wait 4–6 weeks to determine efficacy. May take 4–5 months for complete response.

ANTIDEPRESSANTS

Treatment with antidepressants may be an option for an individual with mild depression; however, they are highly recommended for individuals with moderate to severe symptoms. In addition, for individuals with psychotic symptoms, an antipsychotic would be added. All antidepressants are equally efficacious in treating depression so they are chosen based upon individual treatment response and side effect profiles.

Indications: The antidepressants are the first line of treatment for depression and chronic anxiety disorders. They are chosen based on patient symptoms and individual side effect profiles. For example, more sedating antidepressants would be chosen for depressed individuals with sleep disorders. Table 7–1 shows the major side effect differences among the tricyclics, monoamine oxidase inhibitors, and selective serotonin reuptake inhibitors.

Table 7–1. Comparison of Antidepressant Side Effects

Side Effects	Amitriptyline (TCA)	Fluoxetine (SSRI)	Phenelzine (MAOI)
Anticholinergic	++++	0	+
Sedation	++++	0	+
Hypotension	++	0/+	0
Seizures	+++	0/+	0
Cardiac	++++	0	0
Weight gain	+++	+	+
Sexual dysfunction	++	++++	+++
Other		GI bleeding	Hypertensive crisis

- There are many categories of antidepressants:
  - Tricyclic antidepressants (TCA)
  - Monoamine oxidase inhibitors (MAOI)
  - Selective serotonin reuptake inhibitors (SSRI)
  - Dual serotonin and norepinephrine reuptake inhibitors (SNRI)
  - Norepinephrine dopamine reuptake inhibitors (NDRI)
  - Serotonin 2 antagonist/reuptake inhibitors (SARI)
- *Age considerations:*
  - Children and adolescents respond well to SSRIs and these are considered first-line treatments. However, the FDA warns of a 2% to 3% greater risk of suicidal behavior in children taking antidepressants. This is thought to be due to the delay between early energizing effects of the drugs and delayed improvement in depressed mood.
  - Due to the potential cardiac effects of the tricyclics, these are contraindicated for elderly patients.

Tricyclic Antidepressants (TCAs)

- *Indications:* Depression, anxiety disorders, obsessive-compulsive disorder (clomipramine [Anafranil]), chronic pain (i.e., neurogenic pain, trigeminal neuralgia, diabetic neuropathy, sciatica, fibromyalgia), sleep disorders, insomnia, and cataplexy
- *Mechanism of action:* Tricyclics block the reuptake of serotonin and/or norepinephrine, increasing their availability for neurotransmission. These are desired actions of the drugs. Unfortunately, they also block many other receptors (ACh, histamine, alpha-adrenergic, and sodium channels), causing numerous unwanted side effects.
- *TCA side effects:* Blockade of ACh receptors results in anticholinergic symptoms. Blockade of histamine receptors results in sedation and weight gain. Blockage of alpha-adrenergic receptors causes orthostatic hypotension and dizziness. Blockade of sodium channels can result in cardiac arrhythmias and cardiac arrest, as well as CNS symptoms and possible seizures.
- *Tricyclics still in use* are listed in Box 7–2.
- *Clinical response:* Improvements in energy and sleep may occur within the first 1–2 weeks. Antidepressant effects take 3–4 weeks.
- Because of the potential for severe side effects and even death, TCAs are relatively contraindicated in the elderly, children, pregnant women, and suicidal individuals.

Box 7-2. Some Tricyclic Antidepressants Still in Use

Generic Name	Trade Name
clomipramine	Anafranil
imipramine	Tofranil
amitriptyline	Elavil, Endep, Tryptizol, Laroxyl
nortriptyline	Pamelor, Endep, Aventyl
protriptyline	Vivactil
maprotiline	Ludiomil
amoxapine	Asendin
doxepin	Sinequan, Adapin
desipramine	Norpramin, Pertofrane
trimipramine	Surmontil
dothiepin	Deprimyl, Gamanil
tianeptine	Coaxil, Stablon

Adapted from *Stahl's essential psychopharmacology: Neuroscientific basis and practical applications* (3rd ed.), by S. Stahl, 2008, New York: Cambridge University Press.

Monoamine Oxidase Inhibitors (MAOIs)

- *Indications:* Depression, especially with atypical symptoms such as marked anxiety or phobic symptoms. Because of the potential for serious adverse effects, MAOIs are not considered first-line treatment for depression.

- *Mechanism of action:* Inhibition of the enzyme (MAO) that metabolizes monoamines (serotonin, norepinephrine, dopamine) once they are pumped back into their terminals from the synapse. This increases the availability of monoamine that can be recycled and discharged into the synapse when the cell is depolarized.
- MAOIs include phenelzine (Nardil), tranylcypromine (Parnate), and isocarboxazid (Marplan). In addition, selegiline (Emsam), a longer-acting skin patch, is now FDA-approved for treatment of depression. Other forms of selegiline (Eldepryl) are used to treat Parkinson disease.
- *Clinical response:* Antidepressant effects may take 3 to 6 weeks.
- *Adverse effects and treatments:*
  - Most frequent adverse effects: Orthostatic hypotension, insomnia, weight gain, edema, and sexual dysfunction.
  - Risk for tyramine-induced hypertensive crisis. Avoid foods that are preserved, pickled, or aged (e.g., aged cheese, cured meats or fish, alcoholic beverages). Exception: Low-dose Emsam is not associated with dietary risk. Symptoms of hypertensive crisis may include sudden elevation of blood pressure, severe occipital headache, tachycardia, sweating, fever, and vomiting. Treatment: Hold dose, give medications to block norepinephrine, and decrease blood pressure.
  - MAOIs carry serious risks for drug–drug interactions. Dangerous hypertensive reactions can result from combining MAOIs with drugs that increase adrenergic (NE) levels. These include decongestants, stimulants, antidepressants that increase NE, and appetite suppressants. A possible fatal serotonin syndrome can occur when MAOIs are combined with drugs that increase serotonin. These include SSRIs, TCAs, appetite suppressants with serotonin inhibition, and opioids. When switching from an MAOI to an SSRI, allow a full washout period to avoid serotonin syndrome. Counsel patients to avoid over-the-counter decongestants, St. John's wort, and herbal weight-loss products. These drugs and any other drugs with sympathomimetic qualities can increase the risk of hypertensive crisis.

Selective Serotonin Reuptake Inhibitors (SSRIs)

SSRIs are generally safe and well-tolerated. They are considered the first line of treatment for moderate to severe depression.

- *Indications:* Depression, obsessive compulsive disorder (OCD), panic disorder, social anxiety disorder, posttraumatic stress disorder (PTSD), eating disorders, and borderline personality disorder.
- *Mechanism of action:* SSRIs act by inhibiting the serotonin transport pump. This assures that more serotonin will remain available in the synapse to interact with post-synaptic receptors.
- SSRIs currently on the market include fluoxetine (Prozac, Prozac weekly, Serafem for premenstrual syndrome), sertraline (Zoloft), paroxetine (Paxil, Aropax, Seroxat), fluvoxamine (Luvox, Faverin), citalopram (Celexa, Cipramil), and escitalopram (Lexapro, Cipralex).
- *Clinical response:* The therapeutic effects may take 3 to 6 weeks for depression and 12 to 16 weeks for OCD.

- *Adverse effects and treatments:*
  - Inform parents or guardians of the slightly increased risk of suicidal behavior during the first few weeks of treatment so they can help observe the child's or adolescent's patterns of behavior.
  - As with all antidepressants, observe for a possible swing into bipolar mania, especially in individuals with no prior history of depression. Individuals with a family history of bipolar disorder should be evaluated for additional use of a mood stabilizer.
  - Common adverse effects include anxiety, agitation, akathisia, insomnia, nausea, diarrhea, sexual dysfunction. Most side effects will pass. If akathisia or any other persistently uncomfortable side effect occurs, the individual may need to be switched to another antidepressant. Bupropion (Wellbutrin) can be added to reduce sexual dysfunction.
  - Serotonin syndrome (excess serotonin) results when a person is taking too much of one or more medications that increase serotonin. Observe for symptoms of confusion, extreme agitation, autonomic instability, muscle rigidity, hyperreflexia, hyperthermia, or myoclonic jerking. Symptoms can progress to seizures, coma, brain damage, or death. It is especially important to avoid combining SSRIs with MAOIs. When switching from an SSRI to a MAOI, the washout period should be 2 weeks. When switching from an MAOI to a SSRI, the washout should be 4 to 5 weeks.
  - Serotonin discontinuation syndrome can occur when an SSRI is discontinued abruptly. The symptoms include agitation, nausea, dysequilibrium, and dysphoria. Tapering of the medication is advised.

Other Commonly Used Antidepressants

- *Trazodone (Desyrel)*
  - *Indications* include depression; however, trazodone is very sedating, so it is generally given at night to help with sleep.
  - *Mechanism of action:* Serotonin-2 antagonist/reuptake inhibitor (SARI).
  - *Adverse effects:* There is a slight risk for priapism (painful, prolonged erection) in males.
- *Venlafaxine (Effexor) and Duloxetine (Cymbalta)*
  - *Indications:* Venlafaxine and Cymbalta are used to treat depression and anxiety disorders. In children, venlafaxine is occasionally used to treat ADHD.
  - *Mechanism of action:* These are serotonin/norepinephrine reuptake inhibitors (SNRIs), so they increase the availability of both serotonin and norepinephrine without the widespread side adverse effects seen in the earlier tricyclics.
  - *Desvenlafaxine (Pristiq)* is a newly approved extended release SNRI made from the major active metabolite of Effexor XR.
- *Bupropion (Wellbutrin; Zyban)*
  - *Indication:* Depression and smoking cessation (Zyban). Commonly used as an augmenting agent with other antidepressants, no sexual side effects, useful for smoking cessation. It is sometimes used to treat ADHD in children.
  - *Mechanism of action:* Bupropion is a norepinephrine dopamine reuptake inhibitor (NDRI), so unlike most other antidepressants, it does not target serotonin. Because it doesn't affect one or two specific serotonin receptors, it is the only antidepressant without adverse sexual side effects. It can even cause a reversal of the sexual side effects of the SSRIs when taken in combination.

- *Adverse effects:* Seizures have been reported, so the medication is contraindicated for individuals with a history of seizures or bulimia.
- *Mirtazapine (Remeron)*
  - *Indication:* Depression and anxiety disorders, especially for individuals with anorexia and agitation.
  - *Mechanism of action:* Alpha 2 antagonist/noradrenaline and specific serotonergic agent (NaSSA).
  - *Adverse effects* include the antihistamine effects. Mirtazapine is highly sedating at lower doses and causes weight gain.

ANTIMANIC/MOOD STABILIZERS

An acute manic episode is generally treated with lithium or valproate, or an atypical antipsychotic. If symptoms are inadequately controlled after 10 to 14 days, another first-line medication may be added. The initial goals are to control any unsafe behaviors and decrease symptoms of agitation, irritability, and impulsivity and to return the individual to usual levels of psychosocial functioning. Once stability is achieved, the goals for maintenance are recovery with prevention of relapse and recurrence. Due to the nature of the illness and the side effects of the medications, it is especially important to determine the most effective drug with the least amount of side effects for each individual.

- *Lithium*
  - *Indications:* For acute mania and mood stabilization.
  - *Mechanism of action:* Lithium is a salt. Its mechanism of action is not well understood.
  - *Common side effects and their treatments:*
    - Thirst, nausea, increased urination, fine hand tremor, and gastrointestinal upset:
      - Instruct patients to avoid dehydration, excessive salt or fluid intake. Propranolol and reduced caffeine intake may reduce tremor. Take with meals to reduce GI upset. Avoid NSAIDs due to decreased renal clearance.
    - Other potentially distressing side effects include hair loss, acne, sedation, decreased cognition, and incoordination.
  - Long-term adverse effects on the thyroid and kidneys.
    - Check for family history of kidney disease, diabetes, hypertension
    - Obtain ECG, baseline measures of BUN, creatinine, thyroid; check for pregnancy.
    - Baseline renal function (including BUN and creatinine clearance) should be assessed, and then reassessed every 6 months.
    - Avoid NSAIDs due to reduced renal clearance.
    - Weight gain: Long-term risk for metabolic abnormalities requires monitoring BMI, fasting triglycerides, and other parameters (see metabolic syndrome related to atypical antipsychotic use).
  - *Narrow therapeutic window and risk for toxicity.*
    - Usual adult dosage: 900–1,800 mg/day in divided doses
    - Long half-life yet narrow therapeutic index
    - Narrow therapeutic index requires frequent physical exams and labs. Serum blood levels should be:

- Acute episode: 0.8–1.4 mEq per L
- Maintenance: 0.4–1.0 mEq per L
- *Lithium toxicity:*
  - Prevent toxicity by keeping lithium blood level within the therapeutic window. Polypharmacy with lithium and other mood stabilizers keeps the dosage of lithium lower and reduces the risk for toxicity. Instruct patients to avoid dehydration or excessive salt intake.
  - Seek medical attention at first signs of diarrhea, nausea, vomiting, drowsiness, tremor, muscle weakness, nystagmus.
  - Signs of toxicity include fever, decreased urine output, decreased blood pressure, irregular pulse, ECG changes, and impaired consciousness.
  - Lithium toxicity is a medical emergency. Discontinue lithium immediately. Obtain lithium blood level, electrolytes, BUN, creatinine, urinalysis, CBC, and electrocardiograph. Hydrate. Emesis, lavage, and/or dialysis may be required.
- *Clinical response* in acute mania may take 7 to 14 days.
- Anticonvulsant mood stabilizers
  - *Indications:* For acute mania and mood stabilization.
  - *Mechanism:* Exact mechanisms are not yet known. However, it is believed that the anticonvulsants reduce the flow of ions through ion channels or increase inhibitory (GABA) or decrease excitatory (glutamate) neurotransmission.
  - *Types:* Examples of anticonvulsants that are used as mood stabilizers include valproic acid, carbamazepine, lamotrigine, gabapentin, and topiramate.
  - *Common side effects and their treatments:*
    - Nausea, diarrhea, sedation: Gastrointestinal side effects can be reduced by using the extended-release formulations
    - Weight gain: Monitor weight and BMI; diet and exercise (lamotrigine and topiramate have lowest risk)
    - Tremor: Consider low-dose beta blocker
    - Hair loss
    - Increased risk for thrombocytopenia: Monitor prothrombin time
    - Risk for agranulocytosis (especially carbamazepine): Monitor WBCs
  - *Long-term adverse effects* on thyroid and liver. Obtain baseline and regular measures of hepatic, hematological, and bleeding abnormalities. Check for pregnancy at least every 6 months.
  - *Clinical response:* Therapeutic effects on mania begin after days but mood stabilization may take weeks to months.
  - *Specific differences among the anticonvulsant mood stabilizers*
    - *Valproic acid:* Valproex (Depakote) is available as once-daily dosing. Extended-release formulations (divalproex CR; Depakote ER) are useful for reducing risk of gastrointestinal side effects, and possibly sedation and hair loss. Valproic acid is most commonly used for the acute manic phase and is less effective for maintenance and treatment of bipolar depression.
    - *Carbamazepine (Tegretol):* Second-line augmenting agent for acute mania. Because of risk for agranulocytosis, monitor WBC every 2 weeks for 2 months, then once every 3 months.
    - *Gabapentin (Neurontin):* Well-tolerated but questionably effective for treating mania. Good anti-anxiety and pain control effects.

- *Lamotrigine (Lamictal):* Indicated for bipolar maintenance. Useful for bipolar depression. Risk of rare toxic necrolysis (also called Steven Johnsons Syndrome). Start very low and go slow. Children and adolescents have higher incidence than adults of life-threatening rash.
- *Topiramate (Topamax):* May be a useful adjunct in bipolar disorder. Not considered a first-line treatment. May cause weight loss.

- *Antipsychotic mood stabilizers:* Olanzapine (Zyprexa), quetiapine (Seroquel), and risperidone (Risperdal) have been approved for treatment of acute mania. Olanzapine (Zyprexa) and aripiprazole (Abilify) are FDA-approved for bipolar maintenance. Symbyax, a combination of olanzapine (Zyprexa) and fluoxetine (Prozac), is FDA-approved for bipolar depression.

ANXIOLYTICS/SEDATIVE-HYPNOTICS

Benzodiazepines

- *Indications:* Used to treat anxiety symptoms and some anxiety disorders. Other indications include insomnia, seizures, muscle spasticity, alcohol withdrawal, and induction of anesthesia.
- *Mechanism of action:* Potentiation of the effect of GABA, inhibiting neurotransmission in the limbic system and cortex.
- All benzodiazepines have essentially equivalent pharmacologic actions. Selection is based on time course (onset and duration of effect).
  - Onset of anxiolytic effects:
    - PO: 30–60 min.
    - IM: 15–30 min.
    - IV: 1–5 min.
    - IM and IV available for lorazepam (Ativan), chlordiazepoxide (Librium), diazepam (Valium), midazolam (Versed; used for preoperative sedation and amnesia)
  - More rapid onset is indicated for:
    - Episodic burst of anxiety
    - Falling asleep rapidly
  - Onset of action quickest for diazepam (Valium), lorazepam (Ativan), alprazolam (Xanax), triazolam (Halcion), estazolam (ProSom).
- *Duration of action* is a function of the half-life of the drug
  - Advantages of longer half-lives include:
    - Less frequent dosing
    - Less variation in plasma concentration
    - Less severe withdrawal
  - Disadvantages of longer half-lives include:
    - Drug accumulation
    - Daytime sedation
    - Daytime psychomotor impairment
  - Advantages of shorter half-lives include:
    - No drug accumulation
    - Less daytime sedation
  - Disadvantages of shorter half-lives include:
    - More frequent dosing

- Earlier and more severe withdrawal syndromes
- Rebound insomnia

- *Treatment Implications:*
  - Long-acting benzodiazepines treat more chronic anxiety disorders, seizures, and alcohol withdrawal.
    - Clonazepam (Klonopin): 18–50 hrs
    - Diazepam (Valium): 20–80 hrs
  - Intermediate-acting benzodiazepines commonly treat more acute anxiety symptoms.
    - Alprazolam (Xanax): 6–27 hrs
    - Lorazepam (Ativan): 10–20 hrs
  - Short-acting benzodiazepines treat sleep onset insomnia, and may be used for preoperative anesthesia.
    - Triazolam (Halcion): 1.5–3 hrs
- *Treatment Recommendations:*
  - Use the lowest possible effective dose for the shortest possible period of time.
  - Avoid the desire to increase dosage. Needing a higher dosage is a sign of developing tolerance.
  - Treatment of children and adolescents:
    - As a general approach, begin treatment with a broad-spectrum agent such as a SSRI. Benzodiazepines can be used for acute anxiety and agitation.
    - If ADHD symptoms are also present, adjunctive use of a stimulant or bupropion should be considered.
    - Alpha-agonists such as clonidine (Catapres) and guanfacine (Tenex) should be considered if insomnia, hyperstartle, or hyperarousal symptoms are problematic.
- *Management of Benzodiazepine Side Effects and Discontinuation*
  - *Common side effects:* Drowsiness, fatigue, depression, dizziness, ataxia, slurred speech, weakness, forgetfulness. Advise patients to avoid driving or operating potentially dangerous machines. Stand slowly to reduce dizziness. Patients may be able to adjust the time of the dosage to reduce daytime symptoms.
  - Because of the risk of psychological and physical dependence, long-term use should be carefully monitored. The drugs should be tapered at discontinuation. Instruct patients not to increase the dosage of the drug unless ordered.
  - Discontinuation syndromes depend on the length of time on drug, the dosage taken, the rate of taper, and the half-life. The higher the dose, the shorter the half-life, the more severe the withdrawal symptoms.
  - Withdrawal symptoms include anxiety, nervousness, diaphoresis, restlessness, irritability, fatigue, light-headedness, tremor, insomnia, weakness, risk for seizures and death. Benzodiazepines are cross-tolerant with alcohol, so the withdrawal is similar and very dangerous.

Serotonin Partial Agonists

Buspirone (BuSpar) is an alternative anxiolytic. Buspirone has no risk for physiological dependence. The therapeutic effects may take up to 4 weeks, limiting its use for severe acute anxiety.

Beta Blockers

Propranolol (Inderal) can be useful for reducing peripheral symptoms of anxiety and tremor. It is sometimes used by performers to reduce tremors and individuals with social anxiety to reduce peripheral symptoms. Propranolol can be used for non–anxiety-related tremors such as those resulting from the use of lithium.

Stimulant and Non-stimulant Treatments for Attention Deficit Hyperactivity Disorder

- *Indications for Treatment:*
  - Inattentiveness, impulsivity, and motor hyperactivity
- *Mechanisms of Action:*
  - Two pathways mediate attention, arousal, concentration, and other related cognitive functions: the norepinephrine prefrontal pathway, and the dopaminergic mesocortical pathway. If they fail, inattentiveness and attention deficit may result. We treat attention deficit disorder (ADD) and ADHD by increasing the levels of norepinephrine and/or dopamine with stimulants.
  - Motor hyperactivity and impulsivity are mediated by dopamine activity in the nigrostriatal pathway. In normal individuals, increasing dopamine in the nigrostriatal pathway with stimulants increases motor behavior and impulsivity, whereas patients with ADHD exhibit what may be a paradoxical reduction.
- *Medication Management:*
  - *First-line:* Stimulants (make more DA and/or NE available)
  - *Second-line:* Atomoxetine (norepinephrine reuptake inhibitor [NRI] and antihypertensives (alpha-2 agonists): clonidine or guanfacine. May be first-line for patients with ADHD and tics.
  - *Third-line:* Antidepressants (make more 5HT, DA, and NE available)
- *Stimulants:*
  - The stimulants are considered first-line treatments for ADHD.
  - Tailor the release characteristics to individual needs and response. Of the methylphenidate drugs, the immediate-release compounds last 2 to 4 hours (Ritalin, Focalin, Methylin, Dexadrine), the older sustained-release formulations last approximately 4 to 6 hours (Ritalin SR, Methylin ER, and Metadate ER), and the newer sustained-release formulations offer 8 to 12 hours of benefit (Metadate CD, Concerta, Focalin XR, Ritalin LA) and can be taken once daily.
  - See the list of stimulants in Box 7–3.
- *Side Effects and Nursing Implications:*
  - The most common side effects include headaches, stomachaches, nausea, and insomnia.
  - Stimulants may suppress normal growth; monitor weight and height. May give drug holidays during summer months to allow catch-up from growth suppression. Periodic monitoring of height, weight, blood pressure, pulse, CBC, platelets, and liver function is recommended.
  - Avoid taking stimulants in late afternoon due to potential effects on sleep.
  - Tolerance, dependence, or abuse may develop over time.

Box 7–3. Commonly Used Stimulants for ADHD

Generic Name	Trade Name
d, l-amphetamine	Adderall, Adderall XR
d-amphetamine	Dexedrine, Dexedrine Spansules, Dextro Stat
methamphetamine	Desoxyn
d, l-Methylphenidate	Ritalin, Methidate, Methylin, Attenade
Sustained Release	Ritalin LA or SR, Concerta, Metadate ER or CD, Methylin ER
Transdermal Patch	Daytrana
Dextro isomer only	Focalin, Focalin XR
pemoline	Cylert

Adapted from *Kaplan and Sadock's synopsis of psychiatry: Behavioral sciences/clinical psychiatry* (10th ed.) by B. Sadock & V. Sadock, 2007, Baltimore: Lippincott Williams & Wilkins.

- *Non-Stimulant Treatments for ADHD:*
  - Atomoxetine (Strattera) is a selective NRI that is approved for use in ADHD and is considered a second-line non-stimulant treatment.
  - Bupropion (Wellbutrin) is a weak NRI as well as a weak norepinephrine and dopamine reuptake inhibitor (NDRI). Bupropion is considered a third-line non-stimulant treatment.
  - Other antidepressants that increase norepinephrine (SNRIs, TCAs) have also been used as third-line non-stimulant treatments.
  - Antihypertensives that are used for the treatment of ADHD plus tics, hyperactivity, impulsiveness, and aggression include clonidine (Catapres) and guanfacine (Tenex). The antihypertensives are considered second-line non-stimulant treatments for ADHD.
    - *Side effects and nursing implications:*
      - Side effects may include sedation, headaches, depression, and potentially rebound hypertension.
      - Nursing implications: Monitor blood pressure.

COGNITIVE ENHANCERS FOR DEMENTIA

- *Indications for Treatment:* Cognitive enhancers are prescribed to slow the decline of cognitive function.
- *Acetylcholinesterase Inhibitors:* Early in the course of the illness, ACh inhibitors are thought to enhance memory by slowing down the destruction of ACh.
  - Tacrine
  - Donepezil
  - Rivastigmine
  - Galantamine
  - Side effects of the ACh inhibitors include nausea, diarrhea, vomiting, appetite loss, and increased gastric acid secretion.

- *Glutamate Antagonists:* Excess glutamate may trigger an excitotoxic process with eventual neurodegeneration. Memantine (Namenda) is a glutamate antagonist that appears to have its therapeutic effect by blocking glutamate at one of the glutamate receptors (the NMDA receptor) and stabilizing the neurodegenerative process.
  - Memantine is well-tolerated with few side effects or drug interactions.

MEDICATIONS USED TO TREAT AGGRESSIVE BEHAVIORS

Medications from all of the classes of psychopharmacological agents are used to treat aggressive behavior, a common symptom that can be seen in patients who have any of the mental disorders. First, it is important to try to determine the cause of the aggression and attempt non-pharmacological interventions. If aggression continues and presents a risk to the patient or others, treatments are individualized and can involve the use of any of the following categories of medications: antipsychotics, anticonvulsants, antidepressants, lithium, benzodiazepines, or antihypertensives.

OVER-THE-COUNTER, COMPLEMENTARY, OR HERBAL AGENTS

Some 40% of individuals in the United States use nonprescribed treatments for symptoms of illness. Many of the over-the-counter or herbal supplements are poorly regulated or understood. Some people believe that these supplements are safer because they do not require a prescription; however, that is not necessarily true. Some utilize the same liver P450 enzymes that are used by the other drugs and may therefore cause drug interactions by inducing or inhibiting those enzymes. It is important to educate patients about the potential risks of using nonprescribed drugs.

St. John's wort is a plant-based supplement sometimes used to treat symptoms of depression, anxiety, and sleep difficulties. St. John's wort may cause increased sensitivity to sunlight. Other side effects can include anxiety, dry mouth, dizziness, gastrointestinal symptoms, fatigue, headache, or sexual dysfunction. It can interact with other antidepressants to cause potentially serious side effects. There is not enough research evidence to determine the efficacy of the drug.

The National Center for Complementary and Alternative Medicine at the National Institutes of Health provides information on a variety of complementary and alternative treatments. The best approach is to advise patients to ask their doctor or nurse practitioner before taking any nonprescribed drugs or supplements.

BRAIN STIMULATION THERAPIES

Electroconvulsive Therapy (ECT)

Electroconvulsive therapy (ECT) is a fast and effective alternative treatment for individuals with major depression not helped by medication therapy or who have other serious contraindications for using medication (e.g., pregnancy). ECT increases virtually every neurotransmitter system in the brain. The effects on the noradrenergic system resemble the changes that occur with antidepressant treatment. ECT involves the therapeutic induction of a bilateral generalized seizure. Although generally safe and effective, it is not a first-line treatment for psychiatric disorders due to the invasiveness of the procedure and the side effects. After the seizure induction, EEG shows about 60 to 90 seconds of postictal suppression, followed by the appearance of high-voltage delta and theta waves and a return to preseizure EEG in about 30 minutes. After repeated treatments, it may take 1 to 12 months for the EEG to return to pretreatment appearance. Notable side effects include reversible memory loss and confusion.

Nursing care of a patient receiving ECT may include the following steps:
- Obtain informed consent: Explain and document consent related to beneficial and adverse effects, alternative treatments, natural course of the disorder, and option of no treatment.
- Make sure that the patient remains NPO 6 hours prior to treatment.
- Remove dentures or anything in mouth.
- Establish IV line.
- Insert bite block just before treatment.
- Administer 100% oxygen at 5L per minute during procedure and until spontaneous respiration returns.
- Give an anticholinergic drug to minimize oral and respiratory secretions during the procedure.
- In addition to anesthesia, give a muscle relaxant, as prescribed, to minimize the risk of bone fractures or injuries.
- Observe seizure activity in the foot that has been protected from the muscle relaxant (often a blood pressure cuff is inflated to keep the drug out of one limb).
- Monitor oxygen saturation with pulse oximeter.
- Observe vital signs.
- Observe mental status; patient may be confused and disoriented upon awakening.
- Continue observing at 15-minute intervals.
- After return of gag reflex, patient may resume eating meals.
- Reassure patient that most memory problems will resolve within several weeks.

Transmagnetic Stimulation Therapy

One of the newer treatments for stimulating the brain cells in people with depression who have not responded to other therapies is transmagnetic stimulation therapy (TMS). TMS uses magnetic fields to stimulate the nerve cells. A large electromagnetic coil is placed against the scalp and painless electric currents are produced. Common side effects from the treatment include headache, scalp discomfort, tingling of facial muscles, and lightheadedness. TMS is still considered an experimental treatment and the long-term risks are unknown.

Deep Brain Stimulation

Deep brain stimulation is FDA-approved for treating the tremor associated with Parkinson's disease. Research is underway to determine whether it also might be effective for depression. Deep brain stimulation requires surgery to implant electrodes deep into the brain. Wires from the electrodes are attached to a battery-operated stimulator implanted in the chest (like a pacemaker). Risks include infection, bleeding, delirium, mood changes, lightheadedness, or insomnia. As with TMS, the long-term risks of this treatment are yet unknown.

REFERENCES

American Nurses Association and American Psychiatric Nurses Association. (2007). *Psychiatric–mental health nursing: Scope and standards of practice.* Silver Spring, MD: American Nurses Association.

Institute of Medicine. Committee on Quality of Health Care in America. (2000). *To err is human. Building a safer health system.* Washington, DC: National Academy Press.

Institute of Medicine. Committee on Identifying and Preventing Medication Errors. (2007). *Preventing medication errors: Quality chasm series.* Washington, DC: National Academy Press.

Joint Commission. (2005). *Official "Do Not Use" list.* Retrieved February 17, 2009, from http://www.jointcommission.org/patientsafety/donotuselist/

Sadock, B., & Sadock, V. (2007). *Kaplan and Sadock's synopsis of psychiatry: Behavioral sciences/clinical psychiatry* (10th ed.). Baltimore: Lippincott Williams & Wilkins.

Stahl, S. (2008). *Stahl's essential psychopharmacology: Neuroscientific basis and practical applications* (3rd ed.). New York: Cambridge University Press.

Appendix 7-A. Glossary

Term	Definition
Agonist	Naturally occurring neurotransmitters stimulate receptors and are thus agonists. Drugs that mimic the actions of the neurotransmitters are also agonists.
Antagonist	Substances that block the actions of agonists *in the presence of the agonist.* In the absence of the agonist, the antagonist has no effects. *Example:* Naloxone is an opioid antagonist. It precipitates withdrawal in the presence of opioids, but otherwise has no effect.
Inverse agonist	Drugs that have the opposite actions of their agonists.
Partial agonist	Drugs that stimulate receptors to a lesser degree than the natural neurotransmitter.
Potency	The relative dose required to achieve certain effects. This term is generally applied to the first-generation antipsychotics to describe the relationship between therapeutic dose and side effects. The more potent the drug, the lower the dosage, and the higher the risk of extrapyramidal side effects (EPS). Antipsychotics with low potency tend to be more sedating and have more anticholinergic side effects than the high-potency antipsychotics. *Example:* Haldol (5 mg) is more potent than Thorazine (300–800 mg/d) because less is needed to achieve the same therapeutic effect. Haldol has a much higher risk for EPS. Thorazine is more sedating.

Continued

Appendix 7-A. Glossary (cont.)

Term	Definition
Therapeutic index	The relative measure of the toxicity or safety of a drug and is defined as the ratio of the median toxic dose to the median effective dose. *Example:* The therapeutic index of lithium is quite low and requires careful monitoring of serum levels.
Tolerance	Tolerance is the need for an increased amount of drug to achieve the same effect. It is the process of becoming less responsive to a particular drug as it is administered over time.

8

Treatment Modalities

Elizabeth Arnold, PhD, RN, PMHCNS-BC

Chapter 8 focuses on selected non-pharmacologic treatment approaches designed to improve the mental health of patients. Therapeutic treatment approaches try to help patients use their own mental processes to bring about desired changes, with therapist support. Only nurses with advanced preparation can perform psychotherapy, but all psychiatric nurses should be familiar with relevant treatment models used in psychiatric settings. Interventions with selected special populations and situations, such as domestic abuse, grief, and suicide, are addressed in this chapter.

INDIVIDUAL TREATMENT APPROACHES

Individual counseling in mental health settings represents a goal-directed, theory-based, interpersonal process between a qualified clinician and patient, provided in a skilled, organized way to achieve identified mental health goals. Individual counseling can be provided as a vital component of inpatient treatment, or as a primary form of behavioral treatment in outpatient settings. Most models of individual counseling are time-limited, with a focus on helping patients develop more effective coping strategies.

Patient-Centered Therapy

Carl Rogers developed a nondirective, patient-centered approach, emphasizing patient self-direction, patient responsibility, and a focus on patient strengths. His humanistic model emphasizes the therapeutic relationship between the therapist and the patient, distinguished by the therapist consistently demonstrating empathy, authenticity, and unconditional positive regard for the patient and his or her growth potential.

Rogers believed that the key approach to understanding a patient's issues is reflection. Therapeutic strategies include mirroring what a patient is revealing, and reflecting this understanding back to the patient. This format allows patients to decide what is in their best interest, and to essentially heal themselves.

- *Mirroring:* Tracking the patient's speed, tone, nonverbal expression, and body language, and matching it in the therapist's response. This demonstrates that the therapist is in tune with the patient.
- *Verbal reflection:* Capturing the message of the patient in a fresh new way, and providing this feedback to the patient. By reflecting affect as well as content, the therapist shows empathy.

Psychodynamic Therapy

Psychodynamic therapy is informed by psychoanalytic theory, but differs from psychoanalysis in that it is an interactive treatment modality requiring a therapeutic alliance between the patient and therapist, with face-to-face contact. The focus is on helping patients discover the unconscious motivation from the past driving their maladaptive behaviors in the present, thereby allowing them to make realistic choices that separate the past from the present. Therapy emphasizes exploration of the patient's resistance and expressions of emotion as they occur in the therapy session.

Interpersonal therapy (IPT) is an evidence-based brief form of psychodynamic therapy in which the treatment goal is to improve a patient's interpersonal skills through clarification of feeling states and identifying areas of conflict or dysfunctional patterns of behavior. The emphasis is on working with patients on one or two key issues most closely related to the patient's symptoms and interpersonal deficits. It is based on the premise that corrective action in one sphere of life can have a ripple effect on other aspects of interpersonal functioning. Insight is an important therapeutic factor in the experiential development of more effective interpersonal behaviors. The therapist is active in offering encouragement and support for new behaviors.

Solution-Focused Therapy

Solution-focused therapy is a pragmatic, short-term, strength-based collaborative treatment approach to individual and family issues. The goal of treatment is to enhance effective resolution of problems through cognitive problem-solving and by incorporating the creative use of personal resources and interpersonal strengths as a methodology; the solution lies within the patient and can be accessed with the therapist's support. The solution-focused therapist helps patients think in terms of solutions rather than problems. Strategies the therapist might employ include the use of:

- *Miracle questions:* If someone waved a magic wand and your problem were resolved, what would be different in your life?
- *Scaling questions* ask patients to rate their current perception of the situation, and their progress toward their treatment goals, on a scale of 1 (lowest) to 10 (highest).
- *Exception-finding questions* are based on the premise that bad behaviors do not happen all the time. Asking patients to recall a time when a behavior did not occur broadens a patient's perspective and allows the patient to consider other options.

Cognitive Behavioral Therapy

Cognitive behavioral therapy (CBT) encompasses several different therapies that share some common elements, for example, rational emotive behavioral therapy (Albert Ellis), and cognitive behavioral therapy developed by Aaron Beck (1991).

Cognitive behavioral therapy is an evidence-based, time-limited form of psychotherapy, based on the premise that the way a person perceives and thinks about a situation influences how he or she feels about it and responds behaviorally. Thus, it is not the situation itself, but how a person thinks about it, that creates distress and counterproductive behavior. For example, if a person steps on your foot, your reactions will be quite different depending on whether it was done purposefully or was an accident. Changing thoughts will also change feeling and consequent behaviors.

Beck also believed that people often base their cognitive assessments on basic core beliefs, which were learned early in life. These core beliefs (schemata) continue to color people's thinking patterns throughout life, affecting how they think about themselves and others, if their validity is not challenged.

The goal of CBT is to help patients modify dysfunctional perceptions and corresponding thoughts that negatively affect their emotions and behavior. Cognitive therapy helps people first to identify their maladaptive thoughts, and then to challenge their validity. As people learn to think more realistically, and to change their distorted thinking, they feel better emotionally and this, in turn, affects their behavior in a constructive manner.

Basic Principles and Strategies
- *Cognitive distortions:* Automatic harmful thoughts that people can have in response to stressful situations.
  - *Cognitive triad:* Cognitive distortions related to a person's negative view of him- or herself, the world, and the future. Beck viewed this triad as being influential in the development of depression.
- *Schemas:* Certain ingrained biases or core beliefs that cause people to interpret basically neutral situations in a personalized, negative way. These schemas are shaped by early life experiences and are difficult to dislodge.

Strategies the CBT therapist might use include:

- *Socratic questioning:* Teaching patients to examine their thoughts and to reflect on their potential for having drawn erroneous conclusions through deliberate logical thinking. Socratic questioning makes it possible for patients to think critically about the validity and consequences of their behaviors. Helping patients develop alternative explanations (also referred to as guided discovery) for dysfunctional thoughts makes them better able to come to different conclusions and to devise more realistic solutions to their problems.
- *Cognitive restructuring:* Teaching patients to challenge their irrational beliefs and to substitute positive self-statements for these negative thoughts.
- *Thought-stopping:* Teaching patients to intentionally detach from maladaptive thoughts, setting aside irrational and false beliefs, and using opposing internal self-talk to make self-made rules less absolute.
- *Homework assignments:* Giving patients a homework assignment—a task to accomplish outside the therapy session—reinforces the idea that the patient needs to continue to work on problems between sessions. A mutually agreed-upon homework assignment should be connected with the session agenda. The results of the homework assignment should be reviewed as an early agenda item in each subsequent session.

The therapeutic process for CBT also can include:

- Educating the patient about the CBT model and process of behavioral analysis (antecedents, behavior, consequences).
- Setting an agenda for each session, focusing on a problem identified by the patient for that session.
- Examining core beliefs and cognitive distortions that are feeding the current problem.
- Engaging the patient in Socratic dialogue to test beliefs and challenge dysfunctional thoughts.
- Helping patients learn to monitor their negative automatic thoughts and recognize connections among cognition, affect, and behavior.
- Keeping an activity record or mood check.
- Consistently assessing for changes from baseline.
- Using guided imagery, role-playing, and behavior rehearsal to help patients think about and develop different ways of doing things.
- Coaching and supporting patients in making positive changes.
- Capsule summaries after the agenda is set, and at the end of the session, help patients make cognitive connections between the agenda of the current session and the overall treatment goals.

Cognitive Behavioral Therapy With Children and Adolescents

Many of the CBT strategies used for adults also can be used with school-aged children and adolescents, with consideration given to their developmental level and level of cognitive processing. Children can be taught to recognize unrealistic thought patterns and to assess factual information about the validity of these thought patterns. Putting events in perspective, accepting uncertainties as a part of life, decatastrophizing ("What is the worst that can happen?"), and replacing this with "What could you do to handle this situation?" provides the child with alternative ways of looking at things.

If a child cannot use Socratic questions because of attention, developmental stage, or learning difficulties, it may be possible to learn calming self-talk as a way of replacing negative, anxious self-talk. Referred to as self-instruction training, this can be an effective methodology in helping impulsive children learn self-control skills, and anxious children to reduce their anxiety.

Behavior Modification Therapy

Behavioral therapists believe that all behavior can be modified through systematic manipulation of environmental variables. The focus of behavioral therapy is on measurable behavior, observed in the here and now. Insight, motivation, and past life experiences are not considered in applying behavioral strategies. Behavior modification programs are highly effective for children with developmental disabilities, attention-deficit disorders, conduct problems, phobias, or addictions. They are incorporated as a structural treatment modality in many residential treatment facilities and the juvenile justice system. Behavioral strategies also are used very successfully with adults presenting with anxiety issues.

Treatment outcomes focus on:
• Helping patients create new, more productive patterns of behavior
• Reducing or extinguishing undesired behaviors and behavioral patterns

BEHAVIORAL CONCEPTS AND STRATEGIES

To effectively modify undesired behaviors, it is essential to describe all parts of a particular behavior. Behavioral approaches are based on established principles of learning that can be systematically applied to help patients modify dysfunctional behaviors. Stuart (2009) defines behavior as "any observable, recordable, and measurable act, movement or response" (p. 561). Following a detailed, narrowly focused assessment of a patient's targeted problem, treatment goals are identified, and action-oriented behavioral techniques are employed to help patients achieve them.

Reinforcement

Reinforcement is a key concept in behavioral therapy. Specific reinforcement is used to increase desired behaviors and to decrease undesired behaviors. A reinforcer is defined as anything that increases the probability and frequency of a desired behavioral response, and decreases the frequency of undesired behaviors, when presented as a consequence of a patient's behavior. To be effective, the reinforcement must always follow the target behavior as soon as possible. The reinforcement should fit the targeted behavior, and should be something the patient desires. Using more than one reinforcer is more effective than using only one.
• Reinforcers can be primary in that the reinforcer itself is given as a reward (e.g., candy, food, toy) or they can be secondary (e.g., token economy in which a patient earns tokens or points that can be exchanged for primary reinforcers).

- Reinforcers can be positive (something the person wants) or negative (response the person dislikes, which decreases the probability of the stimulus behavior). Examples of positive reinforcement include verbal praise and giving a child a desired object or activity. Examples of negative reinforcement include withholding of a desired object, activity, or privileges.
- *Premack principle:* Choosing reinforcers or rewards that are meaningful to the patient. Unless the reinforcer has meaning to the patient, it is unlikely that the patient will work for it.
- *Contingency contracts:* Used particularly with children, contingency contracts specifically identify the behaviors requiring change, the conditions under which reinforcement will occur, and any specific time periods for achieving desired behaviors.
- *Token economy:* Reinforcement designed to increase or decrease behavior with the use of tokens, which have no intrinsic value. Patients receive them at the time the behavior is displayed, and can later exchange them for a meaningful object or privilege.
  - Used for children with developmental disabilities, attention deficit/hyperactivity disorder (ADHD), behavioral disorders, and in hospital inpatient treatment and juvenile justice settings.

Schedules of Reinforcement

- Reinforcement schedules (continuous or intermittent) provide direction for how the reinforcers are used to increase desired behaviors. With continuous reinforcement, the reinforcer is given for each expected behavioral response. Intermittent reinforcement is given either based on the rate of the person's response (ratio schedules) or as determined by time factors (interval schedules). A variable ratio reinforcement schedule in which a person is given reinforcement very frequently, and then less frequently as performance improves, produces the highest response rate. The schedules for reinforcement are arranged as follows:
  - *Continuous:* Reinforcement for expected behavioral response is given for every response.
  - *Fixed interval:* Reinforcement is given at distinct time intervals, and a certain amount of time must elapse before the reinforcer is given.
  - *Variable interval:* Reinforcement is provided for the first response after a variable amount of time has elapsed (e.g., 30 minutes).
  - *Fixed ratio:* Reinforcement is given after a fixed number of responses and every nth response is reinforced (e.g., every 5th response).
  - *Variable ratio:* Reinforce after a variable number of responses; the number of responses varies for each reinforcer.
- Extinction is decreasing a behavior by removing rewards that maintain the behavior, such as not laughing when a child misbehaves. The learned behavioral response decreases because it is no longer being reinforced.
- Punishment is inhibiting an undesirable response by making negative consequences contingent upon it (e.g., grounding a teenager).

Other behavioral strategies used in clinical practice include shaping, modeling, and discrimination.

- *Shaping:* Starting with a small component of the desired behavior and gradually adding more parts to a task behavior, like learning a dance routine by adding a few more steps to the combination each time. Initially, the approximations of desired behavior are successively rewarded until the final desired behavior is achieved (successive approximation).

- *Modeling* involves learning a desired behavior by observing competent models performing it, and imitating their behavior. Related strategies include behavioral rehearsal in which a patient practices a new behavior with the therapist, and coaching in which the therapist gives the patient constructive feedback.
- *Discrimination*: Teaching the child or patient to act one way under one set of circumstances, but not in another, by rewarding the behavior response only in the desired set of circumstances.

Behavioral Treatment Sequence

- *Functional analysis:* Collect baseline data, including information about the current conditions under which the targeted behavior occurs (stimulus response chains) and unintentional reinforcement of undesired behaviors.
- State the problem in behavioral terms, as a targeted behavior for intervention.
- Take baseline measures (frequency, duration, stimuli antecedents, specific actions, and consequences).
- Mutually identify behavioral treatment goals in terms of the desired behaviors to be achieved.
- Collaboratively specify concrete actions required to change the maladaptive behavior.
- Jointly connect the reinforcer with performance of the desired behavior.
- Use behavioral strategies (reinforcement, shaping, modeling, discrimination, etc.), to achieve behavioral treatment goals.
- Gradually modify reinforcement schedules from continuous to variable interval or variable ratio as patients improve.
- Monitor changes in behavior from baseline data.

Systematic Desensitization and Flooding

Systematic desensitization and flooding are examples of classical conditioning behavioral treatment methodologies. Both are used as a form of behavioral therapy to help patients cope with unrealistic fears, or phobias.

With *systematic desensitization*, patients are gradually exposed over time to a situation they fear through graded assignments, which are combined with counterconditioning relaxation techniques provided at the same time. The pairing of relaxation with the presence of the feared object or situation allows the associated fear to decrease because it is not possible for a person to be relaxed and fearful at the same time. With practice and over time, patients are able to experience less anxiety when thinking about the feared situation. The imagery is made more intense until patients are able to actively confront their fear in a real-life situation. With therapeutic support and repeated, graded exposure to the actual fearful situation, the patient is gradually able to control the pervasive fear of a previously avoided situation.

Flooding is an accelerated, more intense version of systematic desensitization in which the patient is exposed directly and repeatedly to the anxiety-provoking situation that she or he fears most. By deliberately facing the fear through real-life contact, patients are able to feel confident about their efforts to control their fear response. Therapist support encourages the patient to continue, despite fear.

FAMILY TREATMENT APPROACHES

Having a theoretical understanding of family dynamics and structure is a critical nursing skill for the psychiatric nurse at the basic generalist level. Although psychiatric nurses certified at the basic level are not expected to conduct family therapy sessions, this knowledge forms the basis for comprehensive planning and therapeutic interventions with families of patients, and the family itself as patient.

Families form an important environmental context for mentally ill patients emotionally, and in many instances financially, socially, and politically. Family members caring for adults with persistent mental illness often are called upon to provide substantial caregiving, monitoring their care, and advocating for community mental health services. Responsible informal family caregivers often need support themselves to cope with the sometimes lifetime care that family members with mental illness need to maintain their independence.

Family is defined as a unit consisting of a defined group of people connected by blood and/or emotional ties, who, over time, have developed distinct patterns of interaction and relationship (Boyd, 2007). A family unit can describe two parents and their children, a single-parent family, a same-sex couple or family, step or blended family, common law family, three-generational family units, or a dyad couple without children.

Each family has a unique family history, predictable ways of interacting, and a shared vision of the future. Within each family system are interpersonal *subsystems* of dyads, triads, and so on with defined emotional bonds and common responsibilities. Examples include sibling and spousal subsystems (Friedman, 1998). A *nuclear family* is viewed as a family unit, consisting of a parent or parents and the children living under one roof, and usually related by blood, marriage, or adoption. Example: Mother, father, children living in one household. An *extended family* consists of second- and third-generation relatives (by blood or marriage) of the nuclear family. They may or may not live together or function as a family unit. Examples include grandparents, aunts, uncles, cousins.

Families are dynamic rather than static organisms, and demonstrate a variety of family response patterns ranging from dysfunctional to resilient coping with stressful family situations. In highly stressful situations, family members may need assistance in coping. The role of the nurse is to promote effective family functioning through enhancement of family strengths, helping families to realistically understand and cope with a family member's illness, and linking them with appropriate community supports.

Characteristics of healthy family functioning include:
- Maintaining clear, but permeable boundaries
- Maintaining social integration and collaborative relationships with the community
- Open and honest communication
- Mutually acceptable patterns of:
  - Division of labor
  - Sexual relationship
  - Earning and spending money
  - Parenting skills

THEORETICAL FRAMEWORKS

Family Systems Theory

Family systems theory applies Ludwig von Bertalanffy's systems model to families, viewing the family as a complex, organized, interactive, and holistic organism. Rather than focusing on each separate family member as the phenomena of interest, family theory emphasizes the connectedness and interdependencies occurring among family members. It is how they come together that defines the uniqueness of a family unit. From a family systems perspective, the entire family is viewed as the "patient" so the focus of treatment is on the relationships among family members.

Family System Concepts
- A family system is one in which the organism is more than, and different from, the sum of its parts, and each part mutually influences the others.
- The functioning of each family member is best understood by looking at the family unit as a whole.
- Family values and rules have a tendency to shape individual member behaviors.
- Boundaries differentiate what is included in the family system and what is external to it. They regulate the flow of information into and out of the family.
- The family is conceptualized as an emotional system or unit in which family members are emotionally interdependent and function in reciprocal relationships with one another (Kerr & Bowen, 1988).

A family systems perspective is based on the following concepts:
- *Morphogenesis:* All family systems are in a constant state of change as they adapt to changing family needs.
- *Morphostasis:* All family systems seek stability in the midst of these changes.
- *Homeostasis:* As individual family members change, the family seeks to restore and maintain a steady state of equilibrium or balance.
- *Equifinality:* Family systems can achieve the same goals or outcomes through different routes.
- *Circular causality:* Emotional problems can best be understood contextually, as part of ongoing feedback loops that maintain a problem.

Bowen Systems Theory

Murray Bowen's family systems theory is perhaps the best known framework of family systems therapy. His theory consisted of eight interconnected concepts.
- *Triangles:* A three-person relationship system, which occurs when a two-person system becomes unstable and involves a third party to reduce the tension.
- *Differentiation of self:* Occurs when a person can think reflectively and can stay calm and clear-headed in the face of family conflict rather than responding emotionally.
- *Nuclear family system:* Identifies four relationship patterns—marital conflict, dysfunction in one spouse, impairment in one or more children, and emotional distance between significant family members—that tend to occur when the level of tension rises in a family.

- *Family projection process:* Parents transmit their emotional fears or issues onto one of their children, adversely affecting the child's normal development and behavior.
- *Multigenerational transmission process:* Relationship patterns can be transmitted from generation to generation, so behaviors and emotional issues in one generation will tend to repeat themselves in future generations.
- *Emotional cutoff:* Occurs when people reduce the tension of unresolved emotional issues with family members by reducing or totally cutting off emotional contact with them.
- *Sibling position:* A person's birth order position in his or her family has an impact on individual development and expression. Common characteristics are associated with each birth-ordered sibling position, although children occupying the same position in different families may exhibit differences in functioning.
- *Societal emotional process:* Refers to Bowen's assertion that each of his concepts applied to family therapy also can be applied to larger social groups such as work, social organizations, and society itself.

Structural Family Therapy

The structural model of family therapy, developed by Salvador Minunchin, emphasizes:
- *Family structure:* Interactional patterns that exist within a family (e.g., time spent together, family rules [spoken and unspoken], automatic transactional responses).
- *Subsystems* refer to the subgroups with the family, which are based on generation, gender, or family function (e.g., spousal, parental, sibling subsystems, males or females).
- *Boundaries* refer to the invisible barriers that surround each family subsystem, protecting each from other subsystems and the external world. Boundaries can be diffuse or rigid. In an *enmeshed* family, the boundaries are so relaxed or diffuse that family members become overly involved in each other's affairs. The opposite of an enmeshed family is a *disengaged* family, in which the boundaries are so rigid that family members remain isolated from each other and the larger society.

Structural therapists "join" with the family, mirroring their way of speaking (mimesis). They restructure and reframe family processes to create processes that are counterproductive to the identified pathological ways of relating used within the family.

Strategic Family Therapy

Strategic family therapy, developed by Jay Haley and Cloe Madanes, is based on the premise that symptoms and problem behaviors serve a function in the family system. Strategic therapists maintain that symptoms are also attempts to control a relationship. Change occurs when the therapist works with the family to uncover the interactions that maintain the symptom and change them by creating therapeutic double binds. A double bind clinical strategy provides conflicting messages or directives, so that the message the patient chooses to respond to negates the contradictory message. Such therapeutic strategies include directives or injunctive paradox, in which the therapist might prescribe the symptom. The therapist might also reframe a deviant behavior as being a protective one for the family, or ask an angry family member in denial to pretend to be very angry. Strategic therapists also hypothesize what function a dysfunctional behavior might have for the family. The goal of strategic family therapy is to help family members act in ways that are counterproductive to the problem behavior.

Multi-Systemic Therapy

Multi-systemic therapy (MST) is an evidence-based form of family-oriented, home-based therapeutic services for adolescents ages 12 to 17 who are involved with the juvenile justice system. It works with the family and incorporates a network of interconnected extra-familial community systems (e.g., peer, school, neighborhood) that can provide intervention in one or more settings, using the strengths of each system to facilitate change. The goal is to work with the multiple factors associated with juvenile offenders to decrease behavioral problems and antisocial tendencies. The usual duration of treatment is 4 months, with 60 hours of contact.

The MST program fosters appropriate parental involvement, clear rules and expectations, and behavior change in the adolescent's natural environments of home, school, and neighborhood. The goals of MST are to reduce the incidence of youth arrests and antisocial behavior, reduce substance abuse, reduce the number of restrictive out-of-home placements due to delinquent behavior, and to improve overall family functioning. Treatment is individualized to meet the needs of targeted families through empowering parents to work with the natural network and environment of their children to activate pro-social behavior and social skills.

TOOLS FOR ASSESSMENT

Tools for Family Assessment

The *genogram* is a simple-to-use assessment tool that displays the family history over three generations in a straightforward schematic diagram. Included on the diagram are the ages; dates of marriage, divorce, and death; significant illnesses and mental disorders or chemical dependencies; immigration and geographic moves; occupations; and conflictual or close relationships between family members. Males are represented by squares and females by circles, with ages identified within the square or circle (Varcolis, Carson, & Shoemaker, 2006).

Ecomaps display important relationships occurring between different family members and the larger community-based systems such as work, school, church, or healthcare system. Ecomaps are useful for identifying the intensity and frequency of contact between the family and external resources and other significant people who can provide support for patients and other family members. Lines are drawn from the family members inside the larger family circle to those significant people and institutions with which the family interacts on a regular basis. Straight lines indicate positive relationships, while slashes through the line indicate stressful relationships (Arnold & Boggs, 2007).

Nursing Diagnoses

Planning for family health care necessarily encompasses a knowledge of family social and financial circumstances, and the support networks available to the family. Nursing diagnoses related to the family as a unit, and can include:
- Ineffective therapeutic regime management
- Ineffective family coping
- Ineffective parenting
- Knowledge deficit
- Caregiver role strain
- Ineffective denial
- Complicated grieving

Nursing Interventions

Wright and Leahey (2007) suggest focused interventions designed to identify and build family strengths and improve family problem-solving and coping strategies. These interventions can include:
- Offering information
- Commending family and individual strengths
- Validating and normalizing emotional responses
- Encouraging the telling of illness narratives
- Encouraging respite
- Devising rituals

Other nursing interventions can include promoting self-care for individual family members and the family as a unit, promoting family cohesiveness and supporting family subsystems, reinforcing functional subsystem boundaries, and encouraging open communication.

Health teaching and psychoeducation are particularly important interventions for families, which often assume partial responsibility for their adult mentally ill family member. Referral of the family to National Alliance for Mental Illness (NAMI) and other community networks or agencies for psychological and practical social support is helpful.

Family counseling can be primary interventions or adjunctive to effective child and adolescent individual or group therapy approaches. Encouraging changes in family functioning can have a profound effect on the level and intensity of behavioral symptoms in children. The parent's ability to provide emotional support and appropriate parental monitoring is an important dimension of treatment for most children and adolescents with behavioral or substance abuse problems.

GROUP TREATMENT APPROACHES

Psychiatric nurses participate in and support therapeutic groups with patients. Group therapy was developed as a serious treatment modality for people with mental health issues during World War II, when there were not enough psychiatrists to treat the large number of soldiers requiring psychological assistance. The results were so successful that group therapy was extended to nonmilitary settings.

Types of Therapeutic Groups in Psychiatric Settings

- *Psychoeducation groups* are used to teach patients and/or patient families about specific mental disorders, patient medications, behaviors such as anger management, social skill development, coping information about their mental illness, and vocational skills. Psychoeducation groups in the community can serve as a fundamental source of information about risk factors, crisis intervention, symptoms, treatments, and so on. These groups are usually time-limited and focused on one topic. Typically, they last 2 to 3 hours. Patients learn from each other and often feel freer to ask questions in psychoeducation groups than in one-to-one patient teaching.
  - Family psychoeducation groups are used in inpatient settings to help improve patient outcomes for individuals with schizophrenia, bipolar disorder, and other severe mental disorders. The goal of these groups is to assist families in promoting compliance with medication and successful re-entry of psychiatric patients back into the community. The topics of these groups include information about the mental disorder and co-occurring disorders, if indicated, and the coping skills members will need to provide the appropriate environment for their mentally ill family member.
- *Reality orientation groups* are used with elderly, confused patients. The goal is to help individuals maintain contact with their environment. Props such as calendars, clocks, and common objects are used to stimulate recognition.
- *Resocialization groups* are used with withdrawn, elderly patients or regressed psychotic patients. The goal is to improve the patient's basic social skills by providing patients with an opportunity to establish simple social relationships and to introduce healthy patterns of relating that can be reinforced and strengthened in a group format.
- *Reminiscence groups* are used with cognitively impaired elderly patients who may lack short-term memory, but still have access to long-term memory. A simple object is used to stimulate discussion. A form of reminiscence group is also sometimes used for higher-functioning patients to stimulate life review.
- *Support and/or self-help groups* reinforce the group members' coping strategies and offer practical suggestions. Examples include Alzheimer's disease support groups for family members. Self-help groups, such as Alcoholics Anonymous, provide support for individuals with alcohol or drug abuse as they cope with this difficult disease. In addition to group meetings, individuals can have a "sponsor" from the group be available for support if they experience difficulty between group meetings. Support groups are usually not led by professionals. All nurses should be aware of support groups in their community.
- *Psychodrama* is a highly structured form of group psychotherapy developed by Jacob Moreno in which individual group members can explore, through enacted scenarios, conflictual relationships with significant others. Other group members play the roles of these individuals, and in the process, the subject can experience and clarify issues that otherwise would not be addressed. The format is experiential and enacted in the here and now, as if the situation were currently happening.

- *Activity groups* are the most common type of group therapy for children and pre-adolescents. They take advantage of a child's natural tendency to express feelings through play activities, and their preference to talk about what they are doing rather than about themselves. Activity groups are particularly effective with children between 5 and 12 years of age to help them learn competition, ground rules, getting along with others, goal-setting, and pro-social behaviors.

Group Composition

Group composition is an important component of effective group therapy, and should be intimately connected to a specific group's treatment goals. For this reason, a person who is not a good candidate for one group may benefit from joining a group with different treatment goals. The size of the group is important. Traditional psychotherapy groups function best with six to eight members. Groups with fewer than five or more than eight members do not provide the level of interaction needed for deep exploration of feelings. The following factors are important considerations in group composition:

- Group members must have the capacity to engage in the primary activities of the group, and enough functional similarity to be able to communicate with each other.
- Therapy groups can have a heterogeneous composition, that is a mix of individuals with different diagnoses, or be homogeneous with regard to age, gender, type of emotional problems, personal characteristics, or diagnosis.
- In closed groups, members are identified prior to group treatment, and membership stays relatively constant. Most outpatient psychotherapy groups are closed groups. In open groups, membership fluctuates and group membership can change from session to session (e.g., bereavement groups, psychoeducation groups).

Stages of Group Development

Tuckman (1965) identified five developmental stages applicable to group psychotherapy:

- *Forming stage:* Orientation phase. Acceptance, trust, and inclusion are major group issues. The leader is most active in this stage. Universal norms such as confidentiality, attendance, communication, and rules for participation are addressed.
- *Storming stage:* Control and power issues emerge in the group in the form of testing and acting-out behaviors. Working through these issues helps create an interpersonal climate in which members feel free to disagree with each other.
- *Norming stage:* Group members develop group-specific standards such as disapproval of late members or the level of levity or anger members will accept.
- *Performing stage:* Most of the work of the group related to individual growth, team productivity, and effectiveness takes place during this stage.
- *Adjourning (termination) phase:* Closure for the group as a whole or for individual members takes place during this phase. The task is to review goal achievement and explore feelings about termination at both individual and group levels. Introducing new areas of psychological concern or beginning new initiatives is not appropriate.

Therapeutic Factors

Irvin Yalom (Yalom & Leszcz, 2005) identified 11 curative or therapeutic factors found in successful group therapy.
- The *instillation of hope* occurs when members see other members at different levels of growth and feel they can change, too.
- *Universality* occurs when individual group members realize that they are not alone, and that others have similar problems, thoughts, and feelings.
- *Altruism* occurs when, by helping others in the group, individual members gain more self-esteem.
- As group members talk and share experiences, they can *impart information* previously unavailable to individuals.
- Effective groups offer a safe forum for members to *develop new socialization skills* and are able to correct maladaptive social behaviors through feedback from other group members.
- By *imitating behaviors* of others in the group, members are able to increase adaptive interpersonal skills.
- *Interpersonal learning* occurs as individuals learn from each other.
- *Group cohesiveness* is the sense of belonging, identity, and social acceptance members get from their membership in the group.
- *Catharsis* occurs as members become able to share their pain, successes, and progress achievements.
- *Existential factors* refer to the new sense of personal meaning that people develop through group therapy experiences.
- Groups offer a unique *corrective opportunity to rework earlier family issues* in a new and more productive way.

Group Member Roles

In successful groups, different members typically display task and maintenance functions. These functions are complementary and both are needed for maximum therapeutic effect. Task functions help keep the group focused on the task and directed toward achieving group goals. Maintenance functions help keep the group members connected and interested in working with each other to achieve group goals. Self-functions, also referred to as disruptive functions, occur when individual group members are more concerned about their own agendas than in contributing to or learning from other group members. This can be a form of resistance or the person may simply be unaware of the impact their behavior has on the group.

Task Functions
- Initiating
- Information- or opinion-seeking
- Clarifying or elaborating
- Consensus-testing
- Devil's advocate
- Summarizing

Maintenance Functions
- Encouraging
- Expressing group feelings
- Compromising
- Gate-keeping
- Standard-setting

Disruptive or Self-Functions
- Blocking or diverting discussion
- Power-seeking
- Recognition-seeking
- Dominating
- Attention-seeking
- Clowning or constant joking

Groups for Children and Adolescents

Group therapy formats can be particularly helpful for children suffering from mild to moderate mental disorders or situational crises, such as loss of a parent. Support from peers of similar age and interests offer the most important and influential relationships for this age group. The significance of "peer pressure" that is capable of promoting positive behaviors and encouragement in developing alternative behaviors cannot be overemphasized. Group therapy for younger children focuses on play activities; for school-age children, there is a joint focus on the play activity and talking about it (Varcolis, Carson, & Shoemaker, 2006).

Group therapy for adolescents also can help strengthen the adolescent's ability to resist negative peer pressure in the community by providing constructive feedback about progress or lack of progress, and modeling appropriate responses. Theme-centered groups for children coping with the death of a parent or sibling often offer needed support in schools and other nonpsychiatric settings.

Groups for children and pre-adolescents should be well-structured, with clearly understood but flexible rules and expectations for group member participation. Activities should be consistent with developmentally and age-appropriate expectations. Group discussion can focus on the application of social activity behaviors to group member situations. Seriously disruptive or aggressive children usually are not good candidates for activity groups if they cannot control their behavior well enough to participate and would sabotage group goals.

MILIEU THERAPY

Milieu therapy is a form of therapy that employs the social *environment* of the unit or facility as a primary therapeutic agent. Standard 5c of the *Psychiatric–Mental Health Scope and Standards* (American Psychiatric Nurses Association & American Nurses Association, 2007), in discussing milieu therapy, states that psychiatric–mental health registered nurses provide structures and maintain a safe and therapeutic environment in collaboration with patients, families, and other healthcare clinicians. The term is used to describe a socioenvironmental structure in which the ward or unit functions as a safe, primary therapeutic agent. According to Stuart (2009), the five components of a therapeutic milieu include containment, support, structure, involvement, and validation.

The structure and process of milieu therapy are particularly helpful with conduct disorder in children, addicts, and the seriously mentally ill. Milieu therapy is used in inpatient, partial hospitalization, and rehabilitation settings. Important characteristics of milieu therapy include:
- Planned treatment environment, which acts as a therapeutic agent.
- Communication is open and direct between staff and patients.
- Patients must be willing to actively participate in group activities and decision-making.
- Close contact with community (family, peers, teachers, etc.).
- Enhances reality testing; encourages problem-solving through discussion.

Central to milieu therapy is the use of a therapeutic community in which staff and patients join together to become a unified agent of change and rehabilitation in inpatient psychiatric and addiction centers, psychiatric long-term residential settings, jails, and sometimes shelters.

Therapeutic Community

Pioneered by Maxwell Jones, the therapeutic community is an important component of milieu therapy in many psychiatric inpatient settings. A therapeutic community supports the concept of patient self-governance. Used in a community-based system, the therapeutic community offers practical learning opportunities that are designed to enhance personal development of more effective social skills and social responsibility. The therapeutic community acts as a microcosm of the larger society in which a person is supported through peer influence re-establishing healthy social functioning. Kennard (2004) states:

> The *therapeutic community* is a "living-learning situation" where everything that happens between members (staff and patients) in the course of living and working together, in particular when a crisis occurs, is used as a learning opportunity. (p. 296)

Characteristics of a therapeutic community that incorporate a partial self-governance format for the unit include:
- Daily community meetings in which patients review goals and functional rules, and participate with staff in decision-making regarding issues affecting the hospital unit.
- Patients and staff mutually create the structure, overall guidelines, and social controls needed to maintain a safe, therapeutic environment.
- All clinical activities, including attendance at unit community meetings, treatment groups, job assignments, and other educational or vocational activities, are considered as elements of successful participation in the therapeutic community.
- Privileges, disciplinary pass approvals/disapprovals, and discussion of unit matters needed to maintain the physical and psychological safety of the environment are managed by the therapeutic community as a whole.

ALTERNATIVE, COMPLEMENTARY, AND EXPRESSIVE THERAPIES

Human beings are infinitely complex; therefore, the treatment of individuals with emotional problems and psychiatric illnesses is multifaceted. In approaching patients as bio-psycho-social-spiritual beings, nurses or psychiatric nurses must be open to whatever helps to heal that individual. Alternative therapies such as hypnosis and biofeedback, and expressive therapies of music, play, art, dance, and relaxation are sometimes used in lieu of (or to augment) more traditional approaches to treatment. They can be effective ways to connect with and heal a patient when other approaches fail or cannot be used. A child who cannot speak may be approached with art, music, or dance in addition to play therapy. An individual in a psychotic state can be helped with relaxation techniques or music until the psychosis can be controlled. Anxiety disorders respond to relaxation techniques and the use of art, play, music, and dance to relieve anxious feelings. Expressive therapy works by stimulating the senses and different pathways in the brain. There are special training programs in these types of therapeutic interventions. Adaptability, flexibility, sensitivity, regard for human dignity, a sense of humor, and knowledge of therapeutic needs are all essential components of individuals working with alternative and expressive therapies in the clinical setting.

Relaxation Techniques

Relaxation techniques are behavioral strategies used primarily to assist patients with stress management, performance enhancement, and pain control. They also are used in conjunction with other forms of psychotherapy to reduce anxiety. The simplest form of relaxation techniques emphasizes teaching patients to reduce tension in their body by learning to recognize its presence and then to release the tension or anxiety with special autogenic methods, such as:
- Meditation or centering techniques
- Guided imagery, in which a person mentally visualizes relaxing images or situations
- Progressive muscle relaxation, a method developed by Benson (2000) in which a person tenses then relaxes muscles one at a time, progressively throughout the body
- Deliberate, deep breathing

Relaxation techniques can be accompanied by music or art images and can be used in conjunction with behavioral therapies such as systematic desensitization and biofeedback. Many of these relaxation techniques are used for pain management and in childbirth.

Hypnosis

Hypnosis involves inducing a state of very deep relaxation, which facilitates openness to suggestion and changes in perception (Varcolis, Carson, & Shoemaker, 2006). Some people associate hypnosis with mind control, but this is not the case. People will typically only follow suggestions that would conceivably be within their range of normal behavior. The therapist uses guided relaxation and intense, focused concentration to help a patient achieve a heightened state of awareness, which is referred to as a *hypnotic state* or *trance*. In this state, healing suggestions related to specific tasks or thoughts are given to the patient.

Hypnosis is useful as a form of suggestion therapy for pain control and breaking habits such as smoking or excessive nail-biting. It is also used as an adjunct to psychodynamic therapy to help people uncover painful thoughts and feelings that otherwise would not surface spontaneously. For this reason, hypnosis is sometimes used with treatment-resistant anxiety, phobias, sleep disorders, sexual abuse, and posttraumatic stress disorder.

A caution with the use of hypnosis is that it can sometimes provoke the presentation of false memories. Patients need to be motivated to engage in hypnosis and only a therapist who is clinically trained and licensed to perform hypnosis should use it as a therapeutic technique. Patients with psychotic hallucinations or dissociative disorders would not be good candidates for hypnotic suggestion therapy methods.

Biofeedback

Biofeedback uses electronic equipment to reveal unconscious physiologic processes associated with anxiety, generalized stress, high blood pressure, chronic headaches, certain types of epilepsy, or pain. Biofeedback is used as a complementary mind–body therapy. It is particularly effective as a noninvasive adjunctive treatment for pain. Through a biofeedback unit, which measures such processes as breathing and heart rates, muscle tension, and skin temperature, the patient receives immediate feedback in the form of visual and auditory signals. Types of feedback used are the galvanic skin response, heart rate, blood pressure, temperature, electromyogram (EMG), and electroencephalogram (EEG). The goal of biofeedback is to teach an individual to alter his or her physiological processes from a status suggesting nervous arousal to a state of relaxation. The desired outcome is that the patient will be able eventually to produce the relaxed state associated with a decrease in symptoms without the equipment.

Art Therapy

Art therapy uses an individual's artwork (drawing, painting, sculpting) as a means of communication and expression, rather than relying primarily on verbalization to understand the individual. The artistic creations and the use of color can contain clues or insights into the stressors experienced by an individual. It is the process and the content of the art produced that is important to therapeutic change, not the end product. Art therapy can be appropriate for a wide range of individuals, from sophisticated adults to nonverbal, developmentally delayed children or psychotic patients. It provides an acceptable and controlled outlet for emotions and conflicts that otherwise might remain unexpressed in verbal therapy. The expression of dreams, fantasies, and conflicts through images is encouraged. The goals of art therapy can be ego strengthening, catharsis, uncovering emotions, developing impulse control, and developing an ability to integrate and relate, depending on patient need.

Music Therapy

Music therapy involves listening to music, playing in rhythmic bands, singing, moving to music for relaxation and enjoyment, and getting in touch with feelings evoked when different types of music are heard. Music crosses over many diverse barriers—intellectual, cultural, and linguistic.

Rhythm is the energizer of music. Music integrates the left and right brain hemispheres. It operates at a subliminal level. It is capable of producing a trance-like state, which in turn promotes relaxation and the ability to focus. Music combined with guided imagery is very effective because it continues subliminally where the verbal message leaves off. Music has been used successfully as a distracter for dental patients and people with chronic pain. Music can also be effective with chronically mentally ill and dementia patients.

Play Therapy With Children

Play therapy is a treatment approach rather than an evidence-based treatment modality. It utilizes a child's play as a medium of expression to enhance communication between the child and the therapist. Landreth (2002) suggests that play is a child's language. Children can more effectively express their thoughts, feelings, and what is troubling them through play activities than they can through direct speech.

Play therapy is a particularly useful therapeutic approach for children ages 3 to 12 years. Children can use toys to express feelings verbally and behaviorally in the immediacy of the present, and in a safe environment. Manipulation and positioning of toys and playing games can give the therapist important information about a child's relationships, problems, and ways of coping. Play builds on children's natural inclination to learn about themselves and their environment and provides:

- A safe and natural environment for children to express their feelings verbally or behaviorally.
- Ways to learn social and problem-solving skills and adaptive behaviors, such as taking turns, working out problems, creating your own fun, and getting along with others.
- A medium to uncover clues to the root of the child's problem.

Treatment goals for play therapy include outcomes that help children:

- Experience and express their emotions and concerns in a constructive way.
- Develop respect, self-efficacy, and acceptance of self and others in their environment.
- Develop pro-social and interpersonal skills with school, family, and peers.

Different cultures may have different expectations for play, which need to be taken into consideration with the choice of toys, the setup of the playroom, and the conduct of the play therapy process. Culturally relevant play materials will seem more natural to the child.

Dance/Movement Therapy

Dance therapy is a form of expressive therapy. It involves expressing feelings through the rhythmic body movements of dancing. Rigid, nonverbal, or repressed patients are sometimes able to express through this medium what they cannot express in other ways. Done regularly, it also can be an aerobic exercise with all of the accompanying benefits that such exercise entails. Movement therapy can help both energize and calm with dementia.

CRISIS INTERVENTION

Gerald Caplan (1964), a pioneer in crisis intervention, described crisis as a state that occurs when people are faced with an insurmountable situation or problem and their usual ways of coping are inadequate to deal with the stress. The crisis state is conceptualized as a normal response reaction to an overwhelming, traumatic event. Flannery and Everly (2000) reviews this crisis response as one in which:
- A person's psychological homeostasis is disrupted.
- This person's usual coping strategies are unable to re-establish homeostasis.
- The level of stress associated with the crisis has resulted in functional impairment (p. 119).

Every crisis presents an opportunity for personal growth. The Chinese symbol for crisis has a double meaning: danger and opportunity. Constructive resolution of a crisis can provide a person with stronger coping ability, whereas an inability to resolve a crisis can lead to psychiatric symptoms or personal breakdown. For each person, the goal of crisis intervention is to return the individual to his or her pre-crisis state of functioning.

Characteristics of the Crisis State

When individuals are unable to resolve a significant problem in their lives, they:
- Begin to experience tension and anxiety.
- Experience a decline in their overall functioning and an inability to organize their behavior. As a result, they:
  - Develop somatic complaints.
  - Experience perceptual changes and intense feelings (e.g., sense of urgency, "going crazy," hallucinations).
  - Experience impaired impulse control.
  - Have limited capacity to ask for or draw support from their usual sources of help (support system).

There are three types of crises:
- *Situational:* Specific external event upsets equilibrium, usually occurring at a personal or family level. *Examples:* Cancer diagnosis, job loss.
- *Maturational:* Occurs at transition points in life. *Examples:* Menopause, childbirth.
- *Adventitious:* Accidental, unexpected, usually occurring to larger segments of the population. *Example:* Natural disaster.

Nursing Model of Crisis Intervention

Aguilera (1998) developed a model of crisis intervention in which the presence or absence of balancing factors is a key factor in the resolution of a crisis state. According to this nursing model, an individual, family, or group can experience a biological or psychosocial event that creates a state of disequilibrium and anxiety. If balancing factors are present in the form of realistic perception of the event, adequate situational support, and adequate coping mechanisms, the person will be able to resolve the problem, regain a sense of equilibrium, and the crisis state is averted. On the other hand, if one or more balancing factors are absent, then the problem remains unresolved, the disequilibrium and anxiety continue/escalate, and the person experiences the crisis state.

Crisis intervention treatment focuses on helping patients to create or restore these essential balancing factors so the person achieves his or her pre-crisis level of functional coping.

Phases of Crisis Intervention

Crisis intervention is described as an acute, short-term therapeutic intervention. The goal of crisis intervention is to return individuals in crisis to their pre-crisis adaptive level of functioning and to prevent or reduce the negative effects of the stressors creating the stress. Caplan (1964) believed that the crisis state can be expected to resolve itself in 4 to 6 weeks.

Interventions are focused on an immediate crisis situation or problem that is perceived as overwhelming and traumatic to the individual patient. Because immediate relief is called for, determination of the services and resources needed to return the patient to his or her pre-crisis level of functioning is essential. Support networks can help individuals in crisis begin to function independently.

Assessment and Stabilization Phase

The first priorities in treating a person in a crisis state are to medically stabilize the patient and to ensure the safety of the patient, family, and others in the immediate environment. This requires the nurse to remain calm and in control of the situation, setting limits when needed. Depending on the nature and severity of the crisis state, short-term medication may be indicated. Once the patient is stabilized medically, and is safe, the focus turns to collecting comprehensive assessment data. This is accomplished by gathering specific data about the crisis, that is, concentrating on recent events, what led up to the present state of disequilibrium, the duration of the crisis state, and its impact on others. Data about support systems, previous coping strategies, and the meaning of the crisis to the patient are explored.

Problem-Solving Phase

In the second phase of intervention, it is important that nurses take an active role with patients and families.
- Develop a working alliance with the patient and his or her family.
- Identify and encourage patient strengths and abilities.
- Identify coping mechanisms used successfully in the past.
- Give the patient an opportunity to express emotions; acknowledge fear, anger, helplessness, resentment.
- Help the patient externalize the events of the crisis in a realistic manner.
- Set realistic goals.
- Mutually identify possible solutions, and encourage self-responsibility.
- Help the patient to identify and mobilize social supports and develop new ones.
- Assist the patient, when needed, to make appropriate community support contacts.

Resolution Phase

The third phase of crisis intervention involves helping crisis patients to restabilize their lives and to achieve pre-crisis adaptive functioning. In this phase, the nurse helps crisis victims understand the negative impact of the crisis on their lives, and actively assists them to use their available resources and support networks to resolve the problems at hand and to achieve independent functioning. Successful resolution is evidenced by a decrease in the original presenting symptoms to manageable proportions, satisfaction with the outcome of the crisis intervention, and articulated plans for future action. During this phase, the nurse helps the patient summarize goal achievement and identify healthy ways of coping to prevent further problems. If the patient needs further assistance, or the problems for which the person sought crisis intervention are not resolved to the patient and nurse's satisfaction, referrals for psychotherapy or additional support can be made.

COPING AND ADJUSTMENT

Features of Domestic Abuse and Violence

Domestic violence refers to an escalating, and usually persistent, pattern of abuse in which a person in an intimate relationship controls a vulnerable person or persons through force, intimidation, threat of violence, and/or control of finances. The three most common categories of violence associated with domestic violence involve child abuse, intimate partner abuse, and elder abuse.

Especially vulnerable are children; women ages 16 to 24; frail elders; mentally ill, cognitively impaired, or mentally retarded children and adults; and those with a physical disability. Women are more at risk for abusive behavior, particularly during pregnancy and the period immediately following a separation (Stuart, 2009). Intimate partner abuse in heterosexual relationships tends to be gender-related, with more women being victimized; the majority of spousal or intimate partner perpetrators are men. However, intimate partner abuse also occurs in gay relationships where it is not gender-related: both abuser and victim are of the same sex. Domestic violence is a serious event in which the victim can be killed, physically injured, psychologically traumatized, or neglected. More pregnant women die as victims of domestic violence than from any other cause.

Perpetrators of domestic violence come from all walks of life, socioeconomic strata, educational levels, races, ethnicities, and occupations. They are more likely to have grown up in an abusive household and/or been exposed to community or peer group violence. Most perpetrators have low self-esteem and a dependent personality. They frequently view their victim as their property, and lack impulse control. Poverty, stress, and cultural values supportive of violence as a way of controlling behavior contribute to the development of abusive behaviors. Alcohol and other substance abuse is frequently a precipitating factor, although not the cause of domestic violence.

Types of Abuse
Domestic abuse can take many forms.
- *Emotional abuse* refers to systematic degradation of a person's self-worth in the form of verbal attacks, controlling and/or limiting the victim's rights, isolating the victim from social contacts, and destroying the victim's personal property or pets.

- *Physical abuse* refers to the intentional infliction of bodily harm through punching, beating, kicking, burning, shoving, twisting hair or body limbs, withholding food, or forcing compliance through actual or threatened physical force. Physical abuse also includes denying the victim food, fluids, or sleep.
- *Sexual abuse* is the act of forcing sex on an unwilling person, unsolicited sexual intimacy (fondling breasts or buttocks, or genital contact with no penetration), indecent exposure, and/or forced exposure to sexually explicit material or unusual sex practices. It also includes sexual behaviors with a person who is unable to give valid consent (e.g., a minor, a person with cognitive impairments). Use of a child for pornography or other sexually exploitive activities is sexual abuse. Sexual abuse can consist of not revealing a sexually transmitted disease and failing to take precautions to safeguard the other person. Women with disabilities may be at greater risk. The most common form of sexual abuse of children is *incest*, sex with a family member.
- *Neglect* is the most common form of child and elder abuse. It can be active or passive. Active neglect refers to the intentional disregard for the physical, emotional, or financial needs and welfare of a child, disabled or cognitively impaired adult, or frail elder by caregivers and others. It can include withholding of care or finances, or failure to provide adequate supervision needed by the victim. Passive neglect is not intentional; the caregiver may not be able to provide appropriate care or supervision due to his or her own disability, lack of resources, lack of maturity, or ignorance.

Perpetrators can be paid caregivers or long-term-care personnel as well as family members or persons with legal authority to make healthcare or financial decisions for a victim.

Case Example
Peggy is a 74-year-old widow living alone in the house where she and her husband raised their four children. She has congestive heart failure and has trouble getting around physically. Peggy is pleasant, but intellectually and emotionally limited. Because of her heart condition, she uses only her kitchen, bedroom, and bathroom. Sometimes she eats, sometimes she doesn't. There are always dirty dishes piled up in the kitchen. She can no longer take care of the house and wears diapers, which she discards under her bed. The stench is overwhelming. Although her adult children live in the area, they visit infrequently, and are unwilling (or unable) to see that their mother gets the care she needs. This is an example of passive neglect, which would need to be reported to social services in most states.

The Cycle of Domestic Abuse
There is a predictable cycle to spousal or intimate partner abuse. Without treatment, it always repeats. Articulating this cycle with patient victims can assist the treatment process.
- *Tension building (escalation or buildup) phase:* Tension rises with minor abuses; the victim tries to appease the perpetrator.
- *Explosion (acute battering) phase:* Abuse in the form of physical injury and/or psychological harm occurs.
- *Honeymoon phase:* The abuser is remorseful and apologetic, promising that the abuse will not happen again.
- Later, the tension building phase reappears and the cycle repeats (Dugan & Hock, 2006).

Indicators of Abuse

Abuse should be suspected when injuries are not explainable, family members provide different explanations, or the explanation does not fit the observed injuries. A history of similar injuries, multiple visits to the emergency department, and a delay between the onset of injury and seeking medical care should raise suspicion. While no single injury informs the nurse that physical abuse has occurred, the nurse should look for patterns of injury or more than one indicator related to the possibility of physical abuse.

- *Physical indicators* of abuse can include dislocations, fractures, burns, abrasions on limbs or torso consistent with strap/rope marks, bruising (particularly bilateral bruising to the arms or inner thighs), evidence of repeated bruising without medical cause, or traumatic loss of teeth or hair.
- *Psychological indicators* requiring further exploration with children can include:
  - Sudden changes in school performance
  - Overly compliant, passive, or withdrawn, demanding without reason
  - Running away, or doesn't want to go home
  - Describing the relationship with parent or caregiver as negative
  - Inability to concentrate that cannot be attributed to a physical or psychological cause
  - Reports physical or sexual abuse by a parent or caregiver
  - Refuses to change for gym
- *Sexual abuse indicators* requiring further exploration with children can include:
  - Unusual incidence of urinary tract infections
  - Bruises, itching, rawness in the perineal area or inner thighs
  - Nightmares, fear of going to bed
  - Changes in behavior, extreme mood swings, or withdrawal
  - Unusual interest or highly developed knowledge in sexual matters
- *Indicators of neglect:* Nurses should consider the possibility of neglect when the child or frail elder
  - Is consistently dirty and/or has a distinct body odor
  - Lacks appropriate clothing for the weather
  - Doesn't have lunch or lunch money
  - Lacks adequate medical or dental care, medications, or eyeglasses
  - Appears apathetic, or afraid of something happening to her or him
  - Lack of or inappropriate supervision of a child's leisure, and adolescent sexual activities
  - Abuses alcohol or other drugs
  - Child is frequently absent from school

Mandated Reporting of Child and Elder Abuse

Nurses must follow state laws for reporting child or elder abuse. In most states, professionals are protected from breach of confidentiality in reporting suspected child or elder abuse and neglect. They should inform patients and families of the nurse's report mandates during the initial assessment, or in any case where abuse is suspected. Specific reporting guidelines are incorporated into state laws. In a court of law, the judgment about reporting of child or elder abuse or neglect will be made on the basis of these published guidelines, and what a reasonable and prudent nurse would do in a similar situation.

Treating the Victim
- Treatment begins with the assessment. Interview the alleged victim alone.
- Validate the victim's feelings.
- Document signs of abuse and encourage treatment. (Children entering treatment for depression, anxiety, or eating disorders often have underlying abuse issues, requiring assessment.)
- Children in an abusive situation may need to be removed from the home or placed temporarily with a relative to prevent further episodes of abuse.
- Educate the abused child about self-protective strategies.
- Treatment approaches for children should reflect the child's developmental level.
- Create a safe environment in which the adult victim has safe alternatives should she or he need them (e.g., shelter, staying with a friend or relative).
- Develop a safety plan that details the steps the adult victim should take in case of abuse, including the collection of important papers, money, and phone numbers.
- Educate adult victims about the cycle of abuse, and explore/correct misperceptions that the victim provokes the perpetrator to become abusive.
- Referral to appropriate services for victims and the perpetrator.

END-OF-LIFE CARE

As people live longer and there are more treatment options available for individuals with cancer and other serious medical conditions, mental health issues related to end-of-life take on more relevance.

Kübler-Ross's Stages of Dying

Elisabeth Kübler-Ross (1969), who is well-known for her work with terminally ill patients, identified five developmental stages associated with the dying process. Kübler-Ross's book *Death and Dying* is still considered the classic work in thanatology. Her research findings showed little variation in the basic patterns of individuals, regardless of differences in religious or cultural background. She claimed that most dying patients go through five developmental stages from the time they receive a terminal diagnosis to the time of their actual death. These stages are not prescriptive, as not all patients go through the full sequence of stages. Many people also fluctuate between the different stages, that is, being in denial, getting depressed, bargaining. The five stages Kübler-Ross postulated are:
- *Denial:* "No, not me." The person feels shocked and refuses to believe what is happening. Some people stay in denial throughout their illness, and unless it interferes with appropriate treatment, denial is not necessarily a bad thing. It helps sustain hope for some people.
- *Anger:* "Why me?" As denial subsides and the person acknowledges a terminal diagnosis, anger can emerge. In this stage, patients can be irritable, demanding, critical of others— particularly caregivers, family, even God. As with other forms of anger, it often covers anxiety.
- *Bargaining:* "Yes, me, but…." In this stage, the person tries to strike a bargain with God or the universe, asking for more time, as in "Just let me live until my son graduates."

- *Depression:* "Yes, me." In this stage, the person can experience feelings of hopelessness and helplessness, and can be consumed with the impact of the impending death. The difference between this stage and the acceptance stage is that the person is still working through the finality of death.
- *Acceptance:* "Yes, me, and I am ready." In this stage, the person accepts the inevitability of death, and begins to actively prepare to leave this world. The patient is likely to become more detached from others in the environment and to complete unfinished business.

Dugan (2004) suggests that Kübler-Ross's tireless efforts to portray the human experience of receiving a terminal diagnosis and coping with a significant loss, namely the ultimate loss of self, is largely responsible for the subsequent development of end-of-life care as an important field in medicine today.

Palliative Care

Palliative care recognizes dying as a normal part of the life process. Interventions neither hasten nor postpone death but allow it to proceed as a natural process, and are designed to preserve the highest quality of life for patients. The World Health Organization (WHO, 2002) describes *palliative care* as "an approach that improves the quality of life of patients and their families facing the problems associated with life-threatening illness through the prevention and relief of suffering by means of early identification and impeccable assessment, and treatment of pain and other problems—physical, psychosocial and spiritual."

Palliative care is consistent with a public health approach and is available for all age groups. This type of care addresses the health needs of patients with life-threatening disorders and conditions such as HIV/AIDS, congestive heart failure, cancer, emphysema, neurodegenerative disorders, end-stage diabetes, and renal failure.

Patient comfort is the primary treatment goal of palliative care. The focus of palliative care treatment is on the relief of pain, stress, and symptoms (e.g., shortness of breath, nausea, fatigue, confusion) associated with terminal illness.

Palliative care uses a team approach to address patient and family needs, including pain, management of clinical complications, and modifications to the care plan as the patient's condition changes.

The End of Life Nursing Education Consortium (ELNEC) offers Train-the-Trainer courses for nurses wishing to improve end-of-life care in the United States, administered through American Association of Colleges of Nursing (AACN) and the City of Hope National Medical Center.

Concepts and Practice of Palliative Care
Palliative care should be provided from the time a serious, life-threatening, or terminal diagnosis is given, throughout the trajectory of the terminal illness and actual death, and after the death to help families cope with their loss. Interventions should:
- Be tailored to meet the individualized needs of patients and families.
- Offer professional support, information, and care during the progression of the patient's illness.
- Integrate the physical, spiritual, and psychological components of patient care and support.
- Provide bereavement counseling to families following the death of their family member.

Grief and Grieving

George Engel (1964) describes grief and grieving as a subjective, personal, physical, emotional, and spiritual response to the loss of something or someone important to a person. Although grief is a universal experience, each person grieves in a unique way; there is no single right way to grieve. There is no set timetable for reaching the subsequent stages of grieving, nor are the stages of grief distinct—they overlap and people can revisit previous stages. Intense emotions are normal during the grieving process. Feelings about the loss can come in waves, striking most often when the person is alone or at night.

Bereavement

Bereavement refers to the time following a loss during which a person expresses grief. Persons experiencing loss can include friends and intimate partners, as well as family members. The National Cancer Institute (NCI; using Bowlby's framework) identifies four phases of bereavement that individuals and families experience with uncomplicated grief.

- *Shock and numbness:* Family members find it difficult to believe the death; they feel stunned and numb.
- *Yearning and searching:* Survivors experience separation anxiety and cannot accept the reality of the loss. They try to find and bring back the lost person and feel ongoing frustration and disappointment when this is not possible.
- *Disorganization and despair:* Family members feel depressed and find it difficult to plan for the future. They are easily distracted and have difficulty concentrating and focusing.
- *Reorganization:* When a person dies or a significant loss occurs, there many be several losses, each of which can trigger mental, physical, social, emotional, or spiritual reactions.

Grieving in Children

Children have more problems with grief because of more limited life experiences, concerns about who will care for them, and limited ability to work through their grief verbally. Depending on their stage of development, children may also believe they "caused" the death because of their behavior. Children who experience death or divorce of a parent, especially around the ages of 4 to 6 and 12 to 14, are more at risk for the development of depression later in life.

Grief in children reflects their personality, developmental stage, and meaning of the lost relationship. It is often expressed behaviorally as anger, or avoidance behaviors as if the loss had not occurred. Nightmares, significant changes in eating habits, concerns about their health, school problems, or difficulties in peer relationships can reveal a child's grief. Developmental differences in grieving may reflect the following:

- *Infants and toddlers:* Unaware of the permanence of death, may keep looking for the lost person. May appear unresponsive or lethargic, lose weight or interest in feeding.
- *Preschoolers:* Aware of the physical death, but sees it as reversible. Thoughts about the death may involve magical thinking, including thinking the child contributed to the person's death. Grief gets expressed behaviorally with sleep and eating disturbances, frequent crying or temper tantrums, clinging behavior.
- *School-age children:* Beginning awareness of the permanence of death. May ask questions about where the person goes or what happens after death. School behaviors may reflect aggressive or destructive responses, sudden outbursts, or clinging behavior.

- *Adolescence:* Conceptually aware of the permanence of death. Adolescents express their grief in words and behaviors indicative of losing someone important (e.g., anger, sadness, lack of energy). Loss of a parent during adolescence is difficult because of the adolescent's need to work through transitional period of separation from the parent.

Children should be allowed to attend memorial services, to see the grave site, and to ask questions about the deceased if they wish to do this. They need to have questions responded to honestly in age-appropriate language, and with empathy.

Children need proactive support from the adults in their environment to work though the grieving process, at the time of the loss and periodically during their childhood and adolescence, especially for nodal events such as graduation, starting a new school, or making a move. Some schools have grief groups and peer support for children and adolescents who have lost a significant person in their lives.

Complicated Grief

Most grief reactions are self-limiting and the person begins to integrate the meaning of the lost relationship with having a life beyond the relationship as a necessary part of life's journey. Complicated grief reactions represent extreme reactions to grief in the form of prolonged intense grief or emotional apathy that interferes with functioning. Variables thought to influence the emergence of complicated grief include:
- Sudden, untimely, or unexpected loss
- Suicide or homicide
- Limited social network that the person can call upon
- Significant cumulative losses
- Strong ambivalence (love/hate feelings) toward the relationship
- Overly close, intense relationship

Symptoms of complicated grief include:
- Absence of, or delayed, grief
- Inability to form new relationships
- Persistent feelings about the lost relationship
- Avoiding any reminders of the lost relationship
- Acute anxiety or agoraphobia related to being alone
- Sleeplessness and significant changes in eating habits
- Difficulty carrying out normal routines
- Extended bitterness, numbness, or detachment about life
- Symptoms of depression, anxiety disorders, posttraumatic stress disorder, or substance use disorder related to the lost relationship

Grief therapy is designed to help individuals and families identify and cope with blockages in the grieving process such as unfinished business with the deceased, previous unresolved losses, and insecurity about ability to reestablish relationships without the deceased. Some patients require medication as well.

REFERENCES

Aguilera, D. (1998). *Crisis intervention: Theory and methodology.* Philadelphia: Mosby.

American Association of Colleges of Nursing. (1999). *Position statement: Violence as a public health problem.* Retrieved August 9, 2008, from http://www.aacn.nche.edu/Publications/positions/violence.htm

American Psychiatric Nurses Association and American Nurses Association. (2007). *Psychiatric–mental health: Scope and standards of practice.* Silver Spring, MD: American Nurses Association.

Arnold, E., & Boggs, K. (2007). *Interpersonal relationships: Communication skills for nurses.* St. Louis, MO: W.B. Saunders.

Beck, A. T. (1991). *Cognitive therapy and the emotional disorders.* London: Penguin.

Benson, H. (2000). *The relaxation response.* New York: Harper Paperbacks.

Bowlby, J. (1980). *Attachment and loss, Vol. 3: Loss, sadness and depression.* New York: Basic Books.

Boyd, M. A. (2007). *Psychiatric nursing: Contemporary practice.* Philadelphia: Lippincott Williams & Wilkins.

Caplan, G. (1964). *Principles of preventive psychiatry.* London: Tavistock Publications.

DeRubeis, R. J., & Crits-Christoph, P. (1998). Empirically supported individual and group treatments for adult mental disorders. *Journal of Consulting and Clinical Psychology, 66,* 37–52.

Draucker, C. (2002). Domestic violence: The challenge for nursing. *Online Journal of Issues in Nursing, 7*(1), 2.

Dugan, D. (2004). Appreciating the legacy of Kübler-Ross: One clinical ethicist's perspective. *American Journal of Bioethics, 4*(4): W24.

Dugan, M. K., & Hock, R. (2006). *It's my life now: Starting over after an abusive relationship or domestic violence* (2nd ed.). New York: Brunner-Routledge.

Eimer, B., & Freeman, A. (1998). *Pain management psychotherapy.* New York: John Wiley and Sons.

Engel, G. (1964). Grief and grieving. *American Journal of Nursing, 64*(9), 93–98.

Flannery, R., & Everly, G. (2002). Crisis intervention: A review. *International Journal of Emergency Mental Health, 2*(2), 119–125.

Friedman, M. (1998). *Family nursing* (4th ed.). Stamford, CT: Appleton & Lange.

Gil, E., & Drewes, A. A. (2004). *Multicultural issues in play therapy.* New York: Guilford Publications.

Kennard, D. (2004). The therapeutic community as an adaptable treatment modality across different settings. *Psychiatric Quarterly, 75*(3), 295–308.

Kerr, M., & Bowen, M. (1988). *Family evaluation.* New York: W.W. Norton & Co.

Kübler-Ross, E. (1969). *On death and dying.* New York: Macmillan.

Kwekkeboom, K. (2007). A model for cognitive-behavioral interventions in cancer pain management. *Journal of Nursing Scholarship, 31*(2), 151–155.

Kymissis, P., & Halperin, D. A. (Eds.). (1996). *Group therapy with children and adolescents.* Washington, DC: American Psychiatric Press.

Landreth, G. L. (2002). *Play therapy: The art of the relationship.* New York: Brunner-Routledge.

Landreth, G., Sweeney, D., Ray, D., Homeyer, L., & Glover, G. (2005). *Play therapy interventions with children's problems* (2nd ed.). Northvale, NJ: Jason Aronson.

Lange, S. (2001). *Psychiatric emergencies and nursing actions. Course #925, V2.* Lakeway, TX: National Center of Continuing Education. Retrieved August 28, 2008, from http://www.nursece.com/onlinecourses/925.pdf

National Cancer Institute. (2008). *Loss, grief and bereavement.* Retrieved September 2, 2008, from http://www.cancer.gov/cancertopics/pdq/supportivecare/bereavement.

Rogers, C. (1951). *Client centered therapy: Its current practice, implications and theory.* Boston: Houghton Mifflin.

Stuart, G. (2009). *Principles and practice of psychiatric nursing* (9th ed.). St. Louis MO: Mosby.

Tuckman, B. (1965). Developmental sequence in small groups. *Psychological Bulletin, 63,* 384–399.

Varcolis, E., Carson, V., & Shoemaker, N. (2006). *Foundations of psychiatric mental health nursing: A clinical approach* (5th ed.). St. Louis, MO: W.B. Saunders.

Vickers, A., & Zollman, C. (1999). Clinical review. ABCs of complementary medicine. Hypnosis and relaxation therapies. *British Medical Journal, 319,* 1346–1349.

Wong, D., & Baker, C. (1988). Pain in children: Comparison of assessment scales. *Pediatric Nursing, 14*(1), 9017.

Wright, L. M., & Leahey, M. (2007). *Nurses and families: A guide to family assessment and intervention* (4th ed.). Philadelphia: F.A. Davis.

World Health Organization. (2002). *WHO definition of palliative care.* Retrieved February 1, 2009, from http://www.who.int/cancer/palliative/definition/en/

Yalom, I. D., & Leszcz, M. (2005). *The theory and practice of group psychotherapy* (5th ed). New York: Basic Books.

9

Disease Prevention, Health Promotion, and Education

Elizabeth Arnold, PhD, RN, PMHCNS-BC

Mental health is an integral part of the general health of every individual. In Chapter 9, the focus is on key aspects of mental health promotion and disease prevention. Theoretical frameworks, principles, and strategies associated with patient and professional education are discussed as primary ways to address health promotion and disease prevention both at the individual and community level. Included in this chapter are adult learning principles and developmentally appropriate educational strategies to use with children and adolescents. The chapter identifies important variables that influence teaching and learning.

Disease Prevention and Health Promotion

Disease prevention efforts in mental health are aimed at keeping a mental health disorder from appearing, delaying its onset, stopping or slowing its progression, or minimizing its impact on a person's life. U.S. Surgeon General David Satcher, in his groundbreaking Surgeon General's report on mental health (U.S. Department of Health and Human Services, 1999a), stated, "Americans assign high priority to preventing disease and promoting personal well-being and public health; so too must we assign priority to the task of promoting mental health and preventing mental disorders" (p. 5).

Disease prevention refers to activities that prevent the incidence and reduce the prevalence of mental disorders. Health promotion is conceptualized as a basic human right that emphasizes supporting and enhancing health-related self-management skills needed to achieve maximum functioning and well-being.

Mental health issues of concern range from awareness of personal attitudes toward mental disability, parity, and access to care for behavioral problems in children and adolescents, physical or relationship circumstances with a mental health component, and specific clinically diagnosable mental or addictive disorders.

Preventing the development of mental disorders and/or minimizing their impact on individuals, families, and society through patient and community education is an important health promotion emphasis in today's mental health care arena. In addition to creating a significant emotional and financial burden for these individuals and their families, mental health issues can be extremely costly in terms of reduced or lost productivity because of mental illness. The World Health Organization (2005) estimates that approximately 14% of the global burden of disease is due to neuropsychiatric disorders (NPDs).

Protective and Risk Factors

Because mental health today is considered much more than the absence of mental disorders, education and prevention efforts target social and environmental, as well as personal, variables that affect the development of mental disorders. Often described as risk and protective factors, such variables contribute to an individual's resilience (protective) in the face of challenges to mental health, or increase a person's susceptibility (risk) to developing a mental disorder.

An important goal of health promotion and disease prevention activities is to decrease risk factors and increase protective factors implicated in the development of mental disorders and behavioral problems. *Protective factors* include:
- Social and community supports
- Strength-based competencies
- Knowledge and education
- Culture and spirituality
- Access to care
- Supportive relationships
- Healthy lifestyle
- Safe living environment

Risk factors for mental disorders and behavioral problems represent a complex interplay of biopsychosocial variables. Identifiable risk factors can include:
- Gender, ethnicity, and age
- Lack of access to, or inadequate, health care
- Poverty and homelessness
- Significant losses
- Family history of mental illness or substance abuse
- History of trauma or exposure to violence
- Limited social and financial resources
- Family or marital discord
- Neglect and abuse during childhood
- Weak social ties to the community or cultural group
- Lack of supportive relationships

No one risk factor is responsible for the development of a clinically diagnosed mental disorder (U.S. Department of Health and Human Services, 1999a). Rather, multiple risk factors contribute to the emergence of the disorder, with some risk factors being additive and others being synergistic.

National Resources for Health Promotion and Disease Prevention

Healthy People 2010 presents the health promotion and disease prevention agenda for the nation. This document sets forth health objectives related to preventive health care and identifies outcome benchmarks to verify their achievement. The two overarching goals of Healthy People 2010 involve:
(1) increasing the years and quality of life for all Americans, and
(2) reducing current health disparities.

Specific objectives and health indicators related to tobacco and substance abuse, responsible sexual behavior, mental health, injury and violence, and access to health care are of special interest to the psychiatric nurse. Healthy People 2010 goals and objectives were a principal resource used to develop CDC goals, objectives, and actions.

The Centers for Disease Control and Prevention (CDC) is the nation's premier health promotion and disease prevention agency. The CDC is responsible for tracking actual and potential health problems and morbidity and mortality rates. The CDC takes a holistic view of health, providing guidelines for basic health and wellness and preparedness goals to deal with health hazards and challenges. The CDC (2007) has identified four health protection and promotion impact goals to help focus its work:
• Healthy people at every stage of life
• Healthy people in healthy places
• People prepared for emerging health threats
• Healthy people in a healthy world

THEORETICAL FRAMEWORKS IN PREVENTIVE PSYCHIATRY

Gerald Caplan (1964) is generally acknowledged as the father of preventive psychiatry in the United States. He was one of the first clinicians to adapt public health principles to mental health care and to insist on population-focused prevention as a methodology for preventing mental disorders and promoting mental health. His work in identifying biopsychosocial hazards that contribute to the risk of future mental disorders; his efforts in analyzing the patterns of crisis, which can lead to positive growth or development of symptoms associated with mental disorders; and his insistence on the importance of enhancing competence and social supports as primary prevention strategies were significant forerunners of current primary prevention models.

Health Promotion Model

Nola Pender's health promotion nursing model (Pender, Mudaugh, & Parsons, 2006) takes the position that individuals are willing to engage in health teaching based on their perceptions and beliefs about:

- Their susceptibility to disease
- A disease's severity or consequences
- The potential effectiveness of preventive actions in minimizing health risks

Perceptual health beliefs can differ from individual to individual and affect patient compliance with treatment and making effective lifestyle changes. In general, the stronger the health belief about the severity of a disorder, or the eventual consequences of not taking a particular action, the more likely the person is to engage in health education programs. Pender describes enhancement of the level of well-being and self-actualization of individuals and groups as relevant to health promotion activities. She describes *modifying factors* that can serve as "cues to actions" in encouraging people to engage in health-promoting activities. Cues to action can include interpersonal reminders from friends or family, mass media, and previous experience with the healthcare system and preventive health education.

Social Learning Theory

Albert Bandura's (1977) theory of social learning proposes that *self-efficacy*, defined as the person's perception of his or her ability to perform an action successfully and the belief that such action will have a desirable effect or outcome, is an important correlate of learning behavior. If the person does not feel capable or believes that he or she could not learn the appropriate skills, the person is unlikely to try. The importance of this theory for patient education and related skill development is to break down desired learning tasks into manageable segments that can lead to learner success. When this occurs, the person begins to develop an internal sense of competence (self-efficacy), which stimulates the desire to learn more and to attempt more complex learning tasks.

Bandura described three types of motivators that move people to consider learning new behaviors necessary for their health and well-being:

- Physical motivators, such as memory of previous discomfort or current symptoms
- Social incentives, such as praise and encouragement
- Cognitive motivators, such as perceived self-efficacy and self-determination

Transtheoretical Model of Behavior Change

Prochaska and Velicer's model of behavior change (1997) is particularly useful in helping mentally ill and chemically dependent individuals learn new behaviors that involve a change in lifestyle behaviors currently maintaining the patient's mental health problems. It provides a framework for assessing a patient's readiness to learn, and then matching the educational or treatment program to the patient's state of readiness. This strategy allows the patient more control over the pace of the learning and choosing which behaviors they wish to tackle, and in what order. The stages of change and learning suggestions progress from:

- *Precontemplation:* Patient does not see there is a problem, and is not considering change. *Approach:* Raise doubt, give information to raise awareness of health risk.
- *Contemplation:* Patient sees there is a problem, is thinking about but not committed to changing behavior. *Approach:* Promote discussion of pros and cons of change, give detailed information about possible actions and solutions.
- *Preparation:* Patient sees there is a problem and is willing to make a change within the next 30 says. *Approach:* Help patient choose realistic course of action.
- *Action:* Patient takes concrete actions to make needed changes. *Approach:* Support active steps to change behavior, give feedback, review progress.
- *Maintenance:* Patient perseveres with consolidated actions to sustain positive behavior change. *Approach:* Continue support to sustain progress, accept relapses as temporary, use steps in Preparation phase to resume progress.

Stress Adaptation Model

Gail Stuart's (2009) *stress adaptation model* examines stress from an integrated biopsychosocial perspective. Specific components of her model include:

- *Predisposing factors:* Can be biological, psychological, or sociocultural risk factors such as genetic background, intelligence, age, self-concept, education, financial assets, belief systems, and past experiences.
- *Precipitating stressors:* Stimuli that require additional energy because they are challenging, threatening, or demanding to the person, such as stressful life events, life strains and hassles, or injury. The stimulus is not stressful in itself; it becomes stressful because of the interaction between the self and the stressful situation.
- *Appraisal of the stressor:* Includes a cognitive appraisal of the stressor's impact on a person's well-being. The person mentally and emotionally considers the stressor's meaning, intensity, social attribution, physiological impact, and feelings in evaluating the impact of the stressor.
- *Coping resources:* Includes an evaluation of the person's coping options or strategies related to what the person can do to resolve the stress (financial assets, social supports, knowledge, spiritual beliefs, problem-solving skills).
- *Coping mechanisms:* Refers to efforts directed at stress management. Coping mechanisms can be problem-, cognitive-, or emotion-focused. They can be constructive, in which the individual views the stressor as a challenge, or destructive, in which the individual uses evasion or defense mechanisms to minimize anxiety without resolving the stressful conflict.
- *Continuum of coping responses:* The patient's coping responses are evaluated on a continuum of adaptation/maladaptation, with higher levels reflecting adaptive responses leading to personal growth and well-being and maladaptive responses requiring clinical and/or nursing diagnosis and treatment.

Stuart then identifies nursing goals, assessment focus, direction of nursing intervention, and expected outcomes of care for four different treatment stages. As presented in Table 9–1 below, identifying the treatment stage helps nurses select the most appropriate nursing approaches and activities.

Table 9–1. Treatment Stages and Corresponding Approaches and Activities

Treatment Stage	Treatment Goal	Nursing Assessment	Nursing Intervention	Expected Outcome
Crisis	Stabilization	Risk factors	Environment management	No harm to self or others
Acute	Remission	Symptoms and coping responses	Mutual treatment planning, modeling, teaching	Symptom relief
Maintenance	Recovery	Functional status	Reinforcement and advocacy	Improved functioning
Health promotion	Optimal stage of wellness	Quality of life and well-being	Inspiration and validation	Optimal quality of life

Adapted from *Principles and practice of psychiatric nursing* by G. Stuart, 2009, St. Louis, MO: Mosby Elsevier, p. 53.

PRECEDE-PROCEED Model

The PRECEDE-PROCEED model is a community-based health promotion teaching model consisting of nine phases; the first five relate to the community needs assessment needed to develop the most appropriate teaching program. These data are referred to as the PRECEDE component, and include:

- *Phase 1:* Social diagnosis—people's perception of their health needs and current quality of life.
- *Phase 2:* Epidemiology diagnosis—epidemiology of the health problems in the target population.
- *Phase 3:* Behavioral and environmental diagnosis—specification of the health-related actions most likely needed to change the problem behavior, and systematic assessment of the environmental factors that would influence health outcomes.
- *Phase 4:* Educational and policy diagnosis—assessment of priority factors needing change to initiate and/or sustain desired health outcomes.
- *Phase 5:* Administrative and policy diagnosis—assessment of the actual educational objectives and type of teaching program needed to achieve identified outcomes.

Phases 6 through 9 focus on the logistical, administrative, and evaluative components of the educational program needed to achieve successful educational outcomes, and are the PROCEED component.

- *Phase 6:* Implementation—the process of converting program objectives into the actions to be taken at the organizational level.
- *Phase 7:* Process evaluation—assessment of resources, personnel, quality of practice, and services offered.
- *Phase 8:* Impact evaluation—assessment of intermediate objectives occurring as a result of the training.

- *Phase 9:* Outcome evaluation—assessment of final outcomes in terms of changes in health status, well-being, and quality of life.

The PRECEDE-PROCEED community health promotion education model also identifies predisposing, enabling, and reinforcing factors that influence community education success.
- *Predisposing factors* are previous experience, knowledge, beliefs, and values that can affect the teaching process (e.g., culture, prior learning).
- *Enabling factors* are environmental factors that facilitate or present obstacles to change, such as transportation, scheduling, and availability of follow-up.
- *Reinforcing factors* include the positive or negative effects of adopting the new learned behaviors including social support, fear of recurrence, and avoidance of health risk.

LEVELS OF PREVENTION

Disease prevention activities target three levels of prevention. At each level, education is an essential methodology for achieving health-related goals.

Primary prevention: Actions taken before a mental disorder develops to minimize risk factors and health-related threats to vulnerable populations. From an epidemiological perspective, primary prevention strategies emphasize reducing the incidence of mental disorders. Health teaching focuses on helping patients develop skills and knowledge related to controllable risk factors and promoting a healthy lifestyle. Examples: Parenting classes, stress management programs. In assessing patient learning needs for primary prevention actions, the nurse considers three population levels of primary prevention focus:
- *Universal prevention* strategies target the general public or an entire population group.
- *Selective prevention* strategies target only those individuals or subgroups of a population whose risk factors for developing a mental disorder are significantly higher than that of the general population.
- *Indicated* or *targeted prevention* strategies specifically target those individuals at highest risk for the development of mental disorders.

Secondary prevention: Actions and interventions promoting early diagnosis of symptoms and/or timely treatment near the beginning of a disorder or disease. From an epidemiological perspective, secondary prevention strategies are designed to reduce the number of current cases of mental disorder (prevalence). Examples: Blood pressure screening, depression, or alcohol abuse screening.

Tertiary prevention: Refers to rehabilitation efforts and strategies designed to minimize the handicapping effects of a mental disorder and problem behaviors. (See Chapter 5 on resources for continuing care.) Preventive teaching includes helping patients to cope more effectively with the necessary adjustments that a serious mental disorder imposes. Other tertiary prevention strategies are designed to address challenging behaviors that can be dangerous or disruptive enough to impair education and/or job achievement and quality of life. Supports for rehabilitative efforts in tertiary prevention often are provided through case management.

CULTURAL IMPLICATIONS FOR HEALTH PROMOTION AND WELLNESS

Culturally Sensitive Assessment

In health care, culture is expressed at individual, interpersonal, and community levels related to perceptions of etiology, symptom expression, and treatment expectations. Recommended standards for culturally and linguistically appropriate healthcare services have been published by the Department of Health and Human Services (2001). Psychiatric nurses should be aware of the following cultural differences in meaning about mental illness and treatment in assessing patient learning needs and in planning appropriate health teaching interventions:

- Level of involvement with:
  - Formal healthcare systems
  - Traditional healers and healing rituals
- Meaning of mental health symptoms related to cultural norms
- Patient understanding and acceptance of biomedical model of prescription
- Use of alternative forms of healing
- Impact of political/access factors on health practices
- Implications for taking meds
- Self-awareness of personal cultural heritage and belief systems

Treatment Formats

When constructing the most appropriate treatment formats for culturally diverse patients, psychiatric nurses need to take into consideration:

- The patient's language, ease of oral and written expression
- Differences in affective expression
- Meaning of nonverbal symbols, tone of voice, gestures, physical space
- Family structure, gender differences
- Health beliefs and practices
- Rituals, particularly around births, deaths
- Religious practices and beliefs
- Level of self-disclosure permitted by culture
- Behavioral etiquette and taboo topics
- Social class distinctions

Learn Model for Use With Culturally Diverse Patients and Their Families

L = Listen with empathy
E = Explain your perceptions of the patient's problem
A = Acknowledge similarities and differences in perceptions
R = Recommend treatment
N = Negotiate treatment

Use of Interpreters

Nurses should learn simple words in the patient's language relevant to the treatment protocols. Often, however, this is not sufficient for patients with little or no fluency in English. There are federal mandates related to accommodation for language differences in the provision of culturally competent care. All patients are entitled by law to have an interpreter, if needed, to understand assessment or treatment protocols. Children and family members should not be used as interpreters. Compatibility between the ethnic backgrounds of the interpreter and patient is advised whenever possible, as individuals from different regions in the same country may use different dialects. Guidelines for working with interpreters include:

- Providing the interpreter with a brief summary of the patient
- Explaining confidentiality and limits to confidentiality
- Explaining to the patient the role of the interpreter
- Allowing extra time for the translation and responses, particularly when word interpretation is not enough for understanding
- Explaining to the patient that additional questions may need to be asked for clarification
- Providing opportunities to educate the interpreter about practices and technical terms
- Asking for additional information about nonverbal cues, speech patterns, vocal tone, and other information needed to understand the patient or context of the communication

Spiritual Assessment

The Joint Commission mandates that each person's psychiatric evaluation needs to include an assessment of his or her spiritual needs, the role that spirituality plays in the patient's life, his or her spiritual goals, and what types of supports the patient desires to help cope more effectively with his or her illness. Even with mental illness, people seek to find a purposeful life. Health teaching should incorporate recognition and acknowledgment of spiritual values, especially those that are part of the person's cultural heritage. Teaching interventions that help provide meaning and hope are more likely to be accepted by patients and their families.

SAFETY ISSUES

Joint Commission Standards

The Joint Commission has established 2009 Behavioral Health Care National Patient Safety Goals, which are described on their website (Joint Commission, 2008) as follows:

- *Identify client correctly.* Use at least two ways to identify patients (e.g., patient's name and date of birth). This can be especially important for getting the right treatment and medication to the right patient.
- *Improve staff communication.*
  - Read back spoken or phone orders to the person who gave the order.
  - Create a list of abbreviations and symbols that should not be used.
  - Get important test results to the right staff person quickly.

- Create a step-by-step process for staff to follow when sending a patient to the next caregiver.
- *Use medicines safely.* Create a list of medications with look-alike or sound-alike names, and update the list annually.
- *Check client medications.*
    - Find out what medications the patient is taking, and look for potential interactions between current and any new medications.
    - Provide a list of the patient's medications to the next caregiver and to the patient's primary care physician.
    - Give a list of the patient's medications to both patient and family and provide an explanation of the medications before the patient goes home.
- *Prevent infection.*
    - Follow handwashing guidelines recommended by the World Health Organization or CDC.
    - Report death or injury to patients from infections acquired in the facility.
- *Help clients to be involved in their care.* Help patients and their families understand how to report their concerns and complaints about safety.
- *Identify client safety risk.* Identify those patients who are most likely to commit suicide.

The Joint Commission mandates the reporting of any unexpected occurrence involving death or serious physical or psychological injury. The purpose of identifying unexpected occurrences, referred to as sentinel events, is to reduce their frequency. A *sentinel event* is defined as any unanticipated event in a healthcare setting not related to the natural course of the patient's illness that results in death or serious physical or psychological injury to a person or persons. Examples of sentinel events relevant to mental health settings include medication error, restraint resulting in injury or death, suicide, delayed treatment, and falls resulting in injury or death.

PATIENT EDUCATION

Definition

Patient education refers to any type of planned educational activities developed for the purpose of improving a patient's health status, health-promotion behaviors, health self-management, or well-being. Adults and children learn differently. *Andragogy* is defined as the art and science of educating adults. *Pedagogy* refers to the art and science of educating children.

Patient education is a collaborative, interactive process between nurse and patient in which:
- Instruction and/or skill demonstration is presented formally or informally, depending on the individualized learning needs of the patient and/or family.
- Skill development is based on cognitive understanding.
- Instruction and skill development is developmentally and age-appropriate and culturally sensitive.
- The desired outcome is to produce an observable change in the learner's health knowledge, attitude, and/or behavior related to an identifiable mental healthcare need.

Patient education interventions can focus on:

- Understanding and coping with the disease process itself.
- Increasing medication and treatment compliance.
- Problem-solving and decision-making about coping with the situational and relationship consequences of having a mental disorder.
- Increasing patient confidence in successfully managing day-to-day life experiences through coaching and role-playing.

Understanding the specific learning needs of the learner and the level of the patient's knowledge are all necessary components of effective psycho-education or health teaching efforts.

Domains of Learning

There are three primary domains of learning: cognitive, affective, and psychomotor. The domains are interrelated in comprehensive learning formats. For example, psychomotor practice of skills reinforces and builds on cognitive knowledge. Learning objectives are succinct statements about what the learner should know, be able to do, and how he or she should feel about the issues following the teaching session.

The *cognitive domain* is concerned with content knowledge and the recall or recognition of specific facts. Teaching methodologies to engage the cognitive domain include lecture, discussion, and assigned readings.

In 1984, Benjamin Bloom described six levels of cognitive learning, which are used today, to categorize the level of abstraction of educational objectives:

- *Knowledge:* Recall of information, knowledge of major themes or principles
- *Comprehension:* Able to interpret facts, compare, contrast, and predict
- *Application:* Able to use information, methods, concepts in new situations or applications to solve problems
- *Analysis:* Able to see patterns, connections, and organization of components in order to make inferences, sort evidence, and identify causes
- *Synthesis:* Able to generalize from old ideas to create new ones
- *Evaluation:* Able to compare and discriminate among evidence to make reasoned choices based on sound conclusions

The levels of thinking proposed by Bloom follow a sequential profile. Thus, one must learn new content using the "lower" thinking skills (knowledge, comprehension, and application) before moving on to the more difficult responsibilities of the "higher" thinking processes (analysis, synthesis, and evaluation).

The *affective domain* involves feelings, attitudes, values, and motivation. Attitudes are generally learned more gradually and benefit from a sensitive teacher who actively explores the values and feelings associated with the presented content. The affective domain is the most difficult to measure objectively. Teaching methodologies to engage the affective domain include role-playing, case studies, modeling, and exercises to develop self-awareness.

The *psychomotor domain* involves the use of motor skills and requires practice for mastery. The psychomotor domain focuses on precision of technique, imitation, and manipulation of objects. Teaching methodologies to engage the psychomotor domain include demonstrations, simulations, role-playing, and skills practice. When skills and information are presented at the same time and the learner has an opportunity to practice the skills with immediate feedback, learning is more effective.

Sensory Learning Style Preferences

According to adult learning theory, learners display an input preference for one sense versus another for sending and receiving information. Neurolinguistic programming (NLP), developed by Bandler and Grinder (1975), is based on the premise that people create representational models of the world and use language to symbolize them. This concept can be applied to the teaching–learning process. Listening carefully to the language a learner uses makes it possible to determine if an individual learns better through use of visual, auditory, or kinesthetic (sensory) means. Matching styles of teaching communication (human modeling) to the person's representational system makes it easier for the learner to understand information.

- *Visual learners* respond better to learning environments in which there are written materials, graphic illustrations, electronic slide presentations, or other projected presentations.
- *Auditory learners* search for oral cues, stories, and words to help them learn material. They appreciate having group discussions and an oral presentation of new material.
- *Kinesthetic learners* learn best with hands-on experiences and psychomotor practice. It is easier for them to learn material with demonstrations and when they have an opportunity to role-play or practice a skill. The kinesthetic learner needs to be able to take frequent breaks.

Often it is possible to assess learner style preference by listening to how the person expresses him- or herself in conversation. For example,

- Visual learners may say, "That looks good to me," or "I see what you mean." The visual learner may also look up to the ceiling as if looking for the answers (visual processing).
- Auditory learners may say, "That sounds like an interesting topic," or "I hear what you are saying." The auditory learner may also look toward the side as if listening for the answer (auditory processing).
- Kinesthetic (sensory) learners may appear more active, with movements such as foot-tapping or shaking a leg during a lecture.

Although teaching to a person's preferred learning style is useful, incorporating more than one sense helps most learners retain information better. Learning is reinforced when appealing to several senses, and even more when learners are able to put their learning into practice while receiving feedback.

Readiness to Learn

Individual differences in adult patients' readiness to learn can influence the effectiveness of health teaching. Readiness to learn refers to the learners' willingness to invest time and energy in the learning process because they perceive it as being important. Factors that can influence a person's readiness to engage in a learning process include:

- *Life experiences:* People enter a learning situation with different cultural, educational, and environmental resources to draw from in learning health-related material. Positive experiences can enhance learning readiness; negative experiences can negatively impact learning readiness.
- *Complexity of the learning task:* Self-efficacy and confidence in being able to learn new material enhance learning readiness. When the learning tasks are within the patient's abilities, or can be broken down into smaller, achievable steps, a significant barrier to learning is removed.
- *Language* is an important factor affecting learning readiness if the educator and learner are not equally fluent in the same language. By law, patients who are not able to comprehend health teaching because of language are entitled to have an interpreter. Considering educational and socioeconomic variables that can influence the use and comprehension of language, and framing content with that understanding, are key to the patient learning success.
- *Culture:* Learning topics and presentation that are consistent with cultural beliefs and values boost learning readiness, while those in opposition decrease readiness. Using culturally relevant examples and anecdotes can facilitate acceptance. Patients can be encouraged to share examples from their culture with the nurse. This type of interaction helps to personalize learning and validate the cultural values of the learner.
- *Values, beliefs:* Attitude toward education, self-direction, and beliefs about the capacity to affect health issues through education influence readiness to learn. The cues to action outlined by Pender can be useful in creating teachable moments.
- *Level of anxiety:* High anxiety can compromise the patient's ability to focus attention and comprehend material; mild anxiety can enhance learning. Key to the success of health teaching is reducing a patient's anxiety so learning can take place.
- *Social support* provides motivation and encouragement during the learning process. When family social support is missing, the nurse can and should provide social and educational encouragement during the learning process.
- *Patient's health status:* To learn effectively, people must have the physical strength, endurance, and ability to focus attention. Timing teaching to those periods when the patient has more energy and capacity to focus attention is critical to success.
- *The environment* should also be made conducive to learning, that is, a quiet, well-lit, ventilated space that is free from distractions.

Ability to Learn

Effective teaching plans recognize that one size does not fit all. In addition to assessing patient readiness to learn, psychiatric nurses need to consider the patient's ability to learn.

- *Developmental level:* Personality and cognitive development variables definitively affect learning readiness and ability, but are not always completely correlated with chronological age. Patients at different cognitive and psychosocial developmental levels require different learning strategies to maximize learning. Other factors include cognitive ability and health literacy.

- *Cognitive ability* refers to the extent to which a person can process information. Cognitive factors that can affect the learning process include thought processing deficits associated with schizophrenia, cognitive disorders, and individuals under the influence of psychoactive drugs or alcohol. Learning disabilities, retardation, low reading skill levels, and low health literacy are factors that need special considerations. Without individual accommodations, these individuals will not be successful or motivated to learn new and/or complex material—even if they realize they need to know this information.

Health Literacy

Health literacy is defined as "the degree to which individuals have the capacity to obtain, process, and understand basic health information and services needed to make appropriate health decisions" (Ratzan & Parker, 2006, p. 713). In 2004, the Institute of Medicine issued a landmark Report on Health Literacy, taking the position that health literacy occurs through a combination of education, health services, and cultural factors.

People may be functionally literate, but not health literate. Some of the factors affecting health literacy include:
- Language barriers of either patient or family
- Health topics that are taboo or interfere with strongly held beliefs
- Vocabulary—most instructional materials should be geared to a sixth grade reading level
- Differences between the clinical and human experience of illness

Potential indicators of low health literacy can include:
- Difficulty in engaging fully with the healthcare provider
- Having difficulty explaining medical concerns
- Lack of follow-through with medications, tests, or appointments
- Seldom asking clinically relevant questions, or asking only the general basic questions
- An inability to describe how to take medication, or when to get help

Interventions that promote health literacy include:
- Health materials that are easily readable and contain relevant images and design.
- Using common, simple but concrete terms instead of medical jargon (e.g., telling the patient to take one pill at 8 a.m., and another pill at 8 p.m. is more helpful than telling the patient to take one tablet twice a day)
- Using pictures to illustrate concepts is useful
- Using "teach-back" formats, for example, with dialogue such as, "Let's review the next steps. Could you show me how you would… or how would you know if you were beginning to feel a little manic?"

THE LEARNING PROCESS

Learning is defined as an active and continuous process of acquiring knowledge and skills, manifested by growth and changes in behavior. The goal of health learning is to change behaviors by acquiring appropriate knowledge, skills, and attitudes. With adults, learning is intended to build on life experience, skills, attitudes, and competencies already achieved.

Adult Learning Principles

Malcolm Knowles is recognized as a pioneer in describing the characteristics of the adult learner using principles of andragogy, writing "Adults need to know why they need to learn something before undertaking to learn it" (Knowles, Holton, & Swanson, 2005, p. 64). According to Knowles, adult learners:

- Value self-directed learning
- Are motivated to learn new things that will help them function more effectively
- Want to be active participants in all aspects of the learning process
- Want guidance, but not an authoritarian teaching style
- Want their previous life experiences to be respected as a resource and integrated into their learning process
- Want variety in learning experiences
- Want to be able to immediately apply learning to real-life contexts
- Respond best to pragmatic, problem-centered learning
- Want to learn at their own speed and in their own style

The *learning process for adults* is facilitated:

- When information to be learned has relevance to the learner
- By proceeding from simple to complex content, and from the known to the unknown
- When feedback is given promptly and frequently
- When the learner can test ideas, analyze mistakes, take risks, and be creative
- When the learner has personal knowledge of his or her progress toward the goal
- In situations in which satisfaction is derived
- With recognition and incorporation of the similarities and differences between past experiences and present situations
- When the learner can immediately apply what is being taught
- When individuals are encouraged to integrate their own areas of interest into the learning content
- When learners can assimilate information at their own rate
- When the teacher acts as a guide, but learners are encouraged to find answers to questions on their own

Teaching Older Adults

Older adults may need modification to the learning environment for maximum learning effectiveness. The speed of learning tends to decrease with age, but the depth of learning increases. While it may take people longer to learn as they get older, normal older adults can grasp what is learned at a deeper and more relevant level. Other physical factors should be considered as well to maximize learning, for example, using larger print, making sure the patient has the appropriate hearing aids, and so on (see Chapter 3 for more suggestions).

Some of the strategies that can be used with older adults include:
- Keep explanations brief, but accurate
- Use analogies to illustrate abstract information
- Speak slowly and distinctly
- Minimize distractions
- Use concrete examples in the environment
- Build on past life experiences
- Make information relevant and meaningful
- Present one concept at a time
- Allow time for processing
- Repeat and reinforce information

Teaching Children

Recognizing the child's cognitive and psychosocial stages of development and incorporating this knowledge into a teaching plan are important dimensions of effective health teaching for children. The most effective teaching approaches include describing each behavioral skill, followed by activities that teach and allow the child sufficient time to practice those skills. Role-playing and discussion about choices that allow children to think through options are important components of this form of health teaching for school-age children and adolescents.

In contrast to adult learners, children are much more dependent on the educator for direction. The health educator serves as a role model for the child. Children have much less life experience that can be tapped as a resource for the current learning. They learn more effectively when the presentation is lively and interactive and when the nurse has taken the time to establish a relationship with the child. Games, simple activities, and stories can be used to teach children important concepts about ways to enhance their health and well-being.

Teaching content and presentation should be culturally appropriate and geared to the developmental age of the child (e.g., therapeutic play with puppets or dolls for preschoolers). Pictures and telling stories are useful strategies in helping children explain what they need and how they feel, and engaging them in a learning environment. Diagrams and models can be used to teach school-age children. Children learn best in short sessions, because their focused attention span may be shorter than an adult's. They are eager to learn things, but content must be presented in a concrete, interesting manner and in shorter segments. Children also need consistent, positive feedback to learn appropriate behavior.

Psychiatric–mental health nurses working with children having a clinical or behavioral mental disorder need to be familiar with the Individuals with Disabilities Education Act (IDEA) and Section 504 of the Rehabilitation Act of 1973. These federal laws require that schools provide equal opportunities to succeed in the classroom. Nurses can advise parents of these laws as it will mean that their child, if he or she qualifies, will be eligible for planned special accommodations and individualized behavioral support needed to succeed in the classroom. Test scores, school performance, and parental involvement largely determine eligibility. Children who qualify are entitled to have an individualized education plan (IEP), which mandates and describes the specific teaching accommodations required by the child.

Developing Teaching Plans

A comprehensive teaching plan can help ensure that you have included all necessary content in the allotted timeframe. Teaching plans provide guidelines for the effective implementation of a teaching session. Whether the teaching format represents individual or group instruction, or is presented in a formal or informal way, learner objectives should reflect identifiable nursing diagnoses. Some examples of the North American Nursing Diagnosis Association (NANDA) related to a need for patient education in mental health include:

- Risk for injury or violence
- Noncompliance (with medication or therapy)
- Self-care deficits
- Ineffective individual coping
- Ineffective family coping

It is not possible or advisable to teach patients all they need to know in the increasingly limited time nurses have with patients, thus, it is critical to establish priorities and to differentiate between what is essential and what is nice to know but not critical to treatment goals. In developing a teaching plan for a patient or group, the following should be included:

- Specific patient-focused measurable learning objectives
- Topical outline of content material
- Identification of teaching strategies and learning activities
- Timeframe for planned activities, including time for questions and/or discussions
- Evaluation measurement, using established criteria

While the teaching session should follow the teaching plan, it is important to view health teaching plans as guides or aids to instruction with enough flexibility to allow different delivery methods and learner participation. When standardized teaching plans are used, they should be tailored to the patient's learning needs and abilities. The art of teaching will require that the individualized needs of the learner, some of which may not emerge until the session starts, get fully addressed. Every effort should be made to match teaching strategies with learner developmental levels and individualized needs. Additionally, it is important to view the patient education process as an integral component of the nurse–patient interaction that is not limited simply to the presentation of content or skill development.

Maximizing Teaching Interventions

Structuring the environment to maximize patient learning is essential. The ideal patient teaching environment is one in which the patient feels comfortable, the environment is quiet and private, and the nurse is able to establish a bond with the patient. Using Prochaska and Velicer's (1997) model to determine learning readiness is useful. It also is important to explain why the teaching is important, even if you think the patient knows this already.

When presenting complex material, it is important to:

- Break the material down into manageable chunks
- Deliver key points in sequential order so patients can logically follow the material
- Encourage questions
- Present one idea at a time

- Provide frequent feedback
- Provide opportunities for supervised practice
- Use clear, precise language; many English words have multiple meanings
- Provide transitional cues to help link one set of ideas with another (Arnold & Boggs, 2007)

Incorporating advance organizers can help patients remember complex concepts. A mnemonic is a useful shortcut for remembering unfamiliar terms or concepts. It consists of using letters or familiar words to represent a complex, unfamiliar term or key concept and help the learner remember it. For example, the mnemonic SOAP(IER) helps the nurse remember the important elements of problem-oriented charting (see Chapter 3). At the end of the teaching, the nurse can provide a short summary or ask the patient to provide a summary of what they learned.

Evaluating Patient Teaching

Evaluation of patient teaching should take into account the appropriateness, accuracy, efficiency, and effectiveness of the teaching content and process. Nurses should consider the following in evaluating patient teaching:
- Patient feedback
- Achievement of identified educational outcomes
- If outcomes were not achieved, what needs to be modified
- What went well, what could be improved upon
- What follow-up is needed

The Joint Commission requires documentation of patient teaching, which should include:
- Initial assessment of teaching need and nursing diagnosis
- Teaching interventions linked to nursing diagnosis and the patient's individualized learning needs
- Patient response to teaching interventions
- Additional referrals or modifications of teaching plan

Teaching Strategies for Formal Presentations

- Select a topic of acute interest to you; people rarely forget a presentation by an impassioned teacher.
- Establish clear and measurable goals and objectives for the presentation. Ask yourself, "What do I hope the learner(s) will take from the presentation?" Setting presentation goals and objectives will guide you in planning content and will save preparation time. (A general rule of thumb is that for each 50 minutes of presentation, plan 4 hours for preparation of the material.)
- Complete a literature search and get necessary materials together before developing the content. This will save you time in the long run.
- Organize the material in a systematic fashion; ordering of information increases the ease with which learning takes place.
- Know your audience and gear the presentation to them.

- Select appropriate teaching strategies (e.g., lecture and discussion, case study presentations, role-play, role modeling, seminars, speaker panel, use of relevant examples from clinical practice, gaming/simulation, peer discussions).
- Use a variety of teaching aids (e.g., slides, handouts, simple overhead transparencies, electronic slide presentations, illustrations, audio- and videotapes, chalkboard or dry-marker board, songs, posters). They greatly enhance and complement a presentation and will keep learners actively engaged.

Effective presentations are those in which:
- The purpose of the presentation is clear and consistently demonstrated throughout the presentation.
- The amount of material presented is appropriate to the allotted time.
- The content is related to the learner's abilities and interests.
- Appropriate instructional strategies clearly augment and support the content.
- Learners feel that assignments, content, and presentation are keyed to personal and/or professional goals.
- The environmental climate is conducive to learning (e.g., comfortable temperature, frequent spaced breaks, refreshments, directions to local restaurants, nearby restrooms).
- Written summative evaluations of presenter effectiveness, degree to which objectives were met, and relevance of content to learner needs collected at the end of the presentation are positive and accurate.

Formative and Summative Evaluation of Learning

Two types of evaluation are typically used to evaluate professional learning. The first is the formative evaluation, which is process-oriented. *Formative evaluations* provide ongoing feedback on performance during an educational process as it is actually occurring. The purpose of formative evaluations is to improve or refine a course or educational program. For example, providing formative evaluations about clinical performance at frequent intervals allows nursing students to make performance corrections prior to final evaluation, and to have honest, clear feedback during the learning process.

Formative evaluations given by students to instructors provide information about corrections needed to make instructional materials or presentations more effective and efficient. Formative evaluations typically are internal evaluations to improve program or course content and teaching methodologies.

Summative evaluations provide evaluative information about the results or outcomes of the learning process. They can be completed as an individual process between educator and student, for example, in the form grades and promotion, or as a group process involving numerical ratings. When students evaluate faculty teaching effectiveness at the end of a course or semester, numerical ratings can be used as evidence for tenure, promotion, and merit decisions. It is critical in all summative evaluations, whether of student learning or faculty teaching, that the same consistent, fair, explicit criteria be used to evaluate all faculty and similar program offerings, and that these criteria be uniformly applied. The process and criteria should be known to both the evaluators and those being evaluated.

By contrast with formative evaluations, summative evaluations are given at the end of a course or formal learning process, and are outcome-oriented. Some of the key differences between formative and summative evaluations include:

- Formative evaluations are predominantly prospective and goal-directed toward improvement; summative evaluations are retrospective and focus on achievement.
- Formative evaluations assist with student or program development; summative evaluations assess the quality of student performance or program offerings.
- Formative evaluations provide feedback on a segment of performance; summative evaluations provide evidence of achievement.

REFERENCES

Arnold, E., & Boggs, K. (2007). *Interpersonal relationships: Communication skills for nurses* (5th ed.) Philadelphia: Saunders/Elsevier.

Bacote, J. C. (1994). Transcultural psychiatric nursing: Diagnostic and treatment issues. *Journal of Psychosocial Nursing, 32,* 42–46.

Bandler, R., & Grinder, J. (1975). *The structure of magic I.* Palo Alto, CA: Science and Behavior Books.

Bandura, A. (1977). Self-efficacy: Toward a unifying theory of behavioral change. *Psychological Review, 84,* 191–215.

Bloom, B. (1984). *Taxonomy of educational objectives.* Boston: Allyn & Bacon.

Caplan, G. (1964). *Principles of preventive psychiatry.* New York: Basic Books.

Centers for Disease Control and Prevention. (2007). *CDC's health protection goals.* Retrieved February 3, 2009, from http://www.cdc.gov/osi/goals/goals.html

Center for Mental Health Services. (1998). *Cultural competence standards in managed care mental health services for four underserved/underrepresented racial/ethnic groups.* Rockville, MD: Author.

Institute of Medicine. (2004). *Health literacy: A prescription to end confusion.* Washington, DC: Author.

Joint Commission. (2008). *2009 behavioral health care national patient safety goals.* Retrieved February 3, 2009 from http://www.jointcommission.org/PatientSafety/NationalPatientSafetyGoals/09_bhc_npsgs.htm

Knowles, M., Holton, E., & Swanson, D. (2005). *The adult learner.* London: Butterworth-Heinemann.

National Assessment of Adult Literacy. (2006). *The health literacy of America's adults: Results from the 2003 National Assessment of Adult Literacy.* Retrieved February 3, 2009, from http://nces.ed.gov/pubsearch/pubsinfo.asp?pubid=2006483

Nielson-Bohlman, L., Panzer, A., & Kindig, D. (Eds.). (2004). *Health literacy: A prescription to end confusion.* Washington, DC: The National Academies Press.

Pender, N., Murdaugh, C., & Parsons, M. A. (2006). *Health promotion in nursing practice* (5th ed.). Upper Saddle River, NJ: Prentice Hall.

Prochaska, J. O., & Velicer, W. F. (1997). The transtheoretical model of health behavior change. *American Journal of Health Promotion, 12,* 38–48.

Quinn, F., & Hughes, S. (2000). *The principles and practice of nurse education.* Kingston upon Thames, UK: Nelson Thornes.

Rankin, S., Stallings, K., & London, F. (2005). *Patient education in health and illness* (5th ed.). Philadelphia: Lippincott Williams & Wilkins.

Ratzan, S. C., & Parker, R. M. (2006). Editorial: Health literacy—identification and response. *Journal of Health Communication, 11,* 713–715.

Stuart, G. (2009). *Principles and practice of psychiatric nursing.* St. Louis, MO: Mosby Elsevier.

U.S. Department of Health and Human Services. (1999a). *Mental health: A report of the Surgeon General.* Washington, DC: U.S. Government Printing Office.

U.S. Department of Health and Human Services. (1999b). *Mental health: A report of the Surgeon General. Culture, race, ethnicity supplement.* Rockville, MD: Author. Retrieved February 3, 2009, from http://www.surgeongeneral.gov/library/mentalhealth/chapter2/sec3.html

U.S. Department of Health and Human Services. (2000). *Healthy People 2010: Understanding and improving health.* Washington, DC: Author.

U.S. Department of Health and Human Services. (2001). *National standards on culturally and linguistically appropriate services (CLAS) final report.* Retrieved February 3, 2009, from http://www.omhrc.gov/templates/browse.aspx?lvl=2&lvlID=15

World Health Organization. (2002). *Prevention and promotion in mental health.* Geneva, Switzerland: Author.

World Health Organization. (2005). *Mental health: Facing the challenges, building solutions. Report from the WHO European Ministerial Conference.* Copenhagen, Denmark: WHO Regional Office for Europe.

Other Resources

www.surgeongeneral.gov: Offers reports from the Surgeon General, including landmark reports related to mental health

www.aacap.org: Offers information from the American Academy of Child and Adolescent Psychiatry

www.apa.org: Offers information about stress, anger, coping with trauma, mind-body connections, etc.

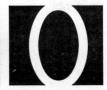

Leadership and Management

Karan Kverno, PhD, PMHNP-BC, PMHCNS-BC

Nursing is faced with many current challenges: the nursing shortage, an aging population, continued health disparities, and increasing social problems such as youth violence. The Institute of Medicine's (IOM, 2001) report, *Crossing the Quality Chasm*, recommended that all healthcare organizations promote health care that is safe, effective, patient-centered, timely, efficient, and equitable. In recognition of evidence on the key role of nurses, the IOM (2004) conducted a study to identify aspects of the work environment for nurses that are likely to have an impact on patient safety, and developed the following goals for transforming the work environment:

- Transformational leadership
- Evidence-based management
- Maximizing workforce capability
- Redesigning work and workspace to prevent and mitigate errors
- Creating and sustaining a culture of safety

ROLES OF A NURSE LEADER

Nursing leadership is essential to promoting safe health care. Leadership roles are available to all nurses who have the knowledge, competence, affiliation, and desire. Most nurses are leaders in one or more aspects of their work. Categories of nursing leadership, described by the

American Association of Colleges of Nursing (AACN, 2007) for the master's prepared clinical nurse leader (CNL), also apply to the psychiatric and mental health nurse:

- Clinician
- Outcomes manager
- Advocate
- Educator
- Information manager
- Systems analyst/risk anticipator
- Team manager
- Member of a profession
- Lifelong learner

Nurse Leader as Clinician

The nurse leader plans, coordinates, integrates, and evaluates patient care. This includes the delegation of nursing tasks, the supervision of the personnel carrying out the tasks, and the evaluation of the outcomes of care. Delegation of nursing tasks to appropriately supervised nursing assistive personnel is one way of addressing shortages in nursing and maximizing workforce capacity. Legal parameters for delegation are specified by state nurse practice acts. In 2007, the National Council of State Boards of Nursing (NCSBN) and the American Nurses Association (ANA) issued a joint statement on delegation that was developed to support practicing nurses in using delegation safely and effectively.

> **Delegation:** The process for a nurse to direct another person to perform nursing tasks and activities.
> **Supervision:** The provision of guidance and oversight of a delegated nursing task.

The NCSBN and ANA (2007) principles of delegation specify that only nursing tasks, not nursing practice, can be delegated. The nurse takes the responsibility and accountability for delegating nursing tasks. Tasks can only be transferred to those individuals with appropriate skill and sufficient knowledge and judgment. Table 10–1 outlines the elements and rights of delegation.

Collaboration. The nurse leader collaborates with the interdisciplinary healthcare team to ensure a seamless transition of care from admission through treatment and back to the community by promoting prompt referrals and timely communication. This may be fostered by including representatives of other disciplines in practice meetings (e.g., conferences, rounds, staff meetings) and by meeting or communicating with alliance groups and referral sources.

Nurse Leader as Outcomes Manager

The nurse leader synthesizes data, information, and knowledge to evaluate outcomes. See Chapter 11 for an overview of outcome evaluation as an ongoing component of evidence-based practice.

Nurse Leader as Advocate

The nurse leader, and all nurses as stipulated by the ANA code of ethics (2001), advocates for and strives to protect the health, safety, and rights of the patient. Nurse leaders advocate for patients by assuring a safe healthcare environment. The rights of the patient, formerly specified by the *Patient Bill of Rights*, are now detailed in a new brochure published by the American Hospital Association (2008) called *The Patient Care Partnership*. Nurse leaders advocate for patients by ensuring that individuals, families, and communities are well-informed and included in healthcare planning. Advocacy can also take the form of working with organizations, such as the National Alliance for the Mentally Ill, on issues relevant to individuals and families with mental disorders. By staying informed of national and local healthcare issues and policies, working on task forces, or voicing concerns to policy-makers, the nurse leader advocates for populations of individuals with mental disorders.

Table 10-1. The Elements and Rights of Delegation

The 4 Elements of Delegation

1. Assess and plan: Based on patient needs and available resources
2. Communicate directions: Include any unique patient requirements and characteristics as well as clear expectations regarding what to do, what to report, and when to ask for assistance
3. Surveillance and supervision: Provide oversight at the level of supervision needed, and clarification as needed
4. Evaluation and feedback: Assess effectiveness and adjust the plan of care as needed

The 5 Rights of Delegation

1. The right task
2. Under the right circumstances
3. To the right person
4. With the right direction and communication
5. Under the right supervision and evaluation

Adapted from *Joint statement on delegation* by the American Nurses Association and the National Council of State Boards of Nursing, 2007, retrieved January 14, 2009, from https://www.ncsbn. org/1056.htm, and *The five rights of delegation* by the National Council of State Boards of Nursing, 1997, retrieved January 14, 2009, from www.ncsbn.org/fiverights.pdf.

Nurse Leader as Educator

The nurse leader uses appropriate teaching principles and strategies to teach patients, precept students, and mentor other healthcare professionals under his or her supervision. Becoming an educator or mentor depends upon having expert knowledge and skills. Brenner (1984) introduced the framework of *"novice to expert"* to describe the process by which novice nurses can develop into experts over time as clinical practice experiences provide opportunities to apply knowledge and develop more proficient skills. Mentoring is an important leadership role that requires, in addition to clinical expertise and knowledge, interpersonal communication skills that inspire and facilitate personal growth.

Nurse Leader as Information Manager

The nurse leader uses information technology systems to utilize current research and provide evidence-based care. The Institute of Medicine's (2006) report *Improving the Quality of Health for Mental and Substance-use Conditions* called for improved technology related to healthcare benefits for improved access to care. Automation of patient-specific clinical information leads to better-organized and retrievable records. In addition, nurse leaders utilize technology to coordinate care between providers and systems.

Nurse Leader as Systems Analyst/Risk Anticipator

The nurse leader participates in the process of continuous quality improvement (QI). High-quality health care is care that is safe, effective, patient-centered, timely, and equitable (IOM, 2001). QI frameworks are called by different names (see below), but the goal is always to assure that quality of patient care is maintained in an organization through an ongoing, continuous effort.

- Quality assurance (QA)
- Performance improvement (PI)
- Total quality management (TQM)
- Continuous improvement (CI)
- Continuous quality improvement (CQI)

Risk managers work to decrease the probability of adverse outcomes related to patient care. They identify patient and organizational risk factors and coordinate corrective actions and strategies to prevent negative outcomes. Continuous QI strategies minimize patient and organizational risk.

Organizational Quality Improvement Frameworks

Organizational quality improvement frameworks are based upon having defined missions and values, professional standards for providers, and guidelines for the provision of care. Two major organizations assist organizations in maintaining safety and quality of care through healthcare accreditation. The Joint Commission (formerly the Joint Commission on the Accreditation of Health care Organizations, JCAHO) accredits behavioral healthcare organizations. The National Committee for Quality Assurance is the leader in accrediting managed care organizations.

- *Mission and Value Statements*
  - Brief statement of the purpose and values of an organization
  - Defines what types of patients are served by the organization
  - Defines the responsibilities of the organization toward the patients
- *Professional Standards*
  - Authoritative statements that include position descriptions, performance skills, and institutional policies
  - An organization's interpretation of a professional's competency
  - Measured through professional outcomes
- *Care Guidelines*
  - Systematically developed (evidence-based) statements to assist in determining appropriate care
  - Institutional protocols and procedures, care plans and pathways
  - Measured though patient outcomes

QI Process

The QI process is a problem-solving process that starts with the assembly of a QI infrastructure. This would include determining the leadership, membership, and meeting structure. To facilitate collaboration, staff involvement is very important. The QI team identifies annual quality goals, outcome monitoring and evaluation processes, and participates in the development of performance appraisals. (See Table 10–2 for facilitators of and barriers to successful QI.)

- *Plan priorities and goals*
  - Define the mission statement and goals
  - What are the patient's expectations?
  - What criteria define quality?
  - What are the expected outcomes of this service?
  - How will outcomes be monitored?
- *Identify processes or services that need improvement and design solutions*
  - Describe current processes, identify data that are needed
  - Localize problems: sentinel events, incident reports, chart audits
  - Conduct a root cause analysis to specify the organizational underlying causes, not just the immediately obvious errors or incidents
  - Generate solutions to root causes and develop a pilot study
- *Measure performance*
  - Test the pilot and collect outcome data
  - Outcome measures may include medication errors, functional outcomes, patient satisfaction, intervention times, or costs per capita
- *Analyze data*
  - Evaluate the pilot data; compare with baseline data
  - Determine whether the change was effective
- *Improve practice*
  - Standardize the new process or repeat the problem-solving process
  - Disseminate the results to the organizational leaders and staff

Table 10–2. Facilitators of and Barriers to Successful QI

Facilitators of QI	Barriers to Successful Change

• Perceived relevance
• Sufficient expertise
• Motivational (transformational) leadership
  - Conveys the importance of QI
  - Organizes educational activities to promote quality
  - Commits resources to support QI program
  - Acts as clinical champion, keeping the team on track
  - Recognizes staff for their QI efforts
  - Institutionalizes QI
  - Demonstrates program successes
  - Shares outcomes with staff
	• Lack of system support
	• Lack of financial resources
	• Lack of time
	• Conflicting organizational goals
	• Insufficient expertise
	• Information overload
	• Lack of understanding regarding purpose
	• Lack of feedback to staff

Nurse Leader as Team Manager

The nurse leader is able to properly delegate and manage the nursing team resources (human and fiscal) and serve as a leader and partner in the interdisciplinary healthcare team. *Resource utilization* is a standard of psychiatric–mental health nursing practice that is defined by the consideration of factors relating to safety, effectiveness, and cost in planning and delivering patient care. Managerial roles include:

- *Staffing:* Chooses the management structure, coordinating people, time, task assignments
- *Recruiting:* Hiring, training, scheduling, ongoing staff development
- *Planning:* Defining goals, objectives, policies, procedures, resource allocation
- *Conducting:* Performance evaluations, analyzing financial activities, monitoring quality of care
- *Supervising:* Directing, guiding, and influencing an individual's performance

LEADERSHIP STYLE

Good leader attributes include being consistent, responsible, calm, articulate, and organized. The best leadership style depends upon the setting, the expertise of the staff, and the needs of the organization. The following is a description of different styles of leadership:

- *Autocratic*
  - Leader retains all authority, makes all decisions, and establishes one-way communication with the work group
  - Can be effective in crisis situations
- *Democratic*
  - Leader focuses on teamwork and workgroup participation in decision-making
  - Leader collaborates with others in making decisions
  - Can be effective with mature staff
- *Laissez-Faire*
  - Leader gives up control with free-run or permissive style
  - Can only be effective with highly motivated staff
- *Situational*
  - The situation is the major determinant of the leader's behaviors
  - Flexible adaptation to needs of individual or work group
  - Directing: More important with new staff
  - Coaching: For those who are more experienced but still need some guidance
  - Supporting: Assists in problem-solving
  - Delegating: Transfers responsibility while retaining accountability; promotes staff development
- *Transformational*
  - Leader inspires and motivates others to follow
  - Leader has vision, passion, enthusiasm, and energy
  - Leader creates and communicates shared vision and values
  - Leader champions solutions to patient and organizational challenges
  - Leader provides intellectual stimulation

LEADERSHIP POWER

Leaders have power that allows them to accomplish goals. Marquis and Huston (1992) describe the following types of nursing leadership power:

- *Reward:* Power obtained by the ability to grant favors or reward others with whatever they value
- *Coercive:* Power based on a person's real or perceived fear of punishment by another person
- *Legitimate:* Power derived from a person's organizational title or position rather than from a personal quality
- *Expert:* Power gained through knowledge, expertise, or experience
- *Referent:* Power given by others because the leader is perceived as powerful
- *Informational:* Power that results when one person has, or is perceived to have, special information that another desires

CONFLICT RESOLUTION SKILLS

Leaders need conflict resolution skills to foster healthy communication among staff. Staff members may present interpersonal conflicts to the leader. Before attempting any conflict resolution strategies, the leader needs to know his or her own role and response to conflict, and manage any uncomfortable feelings. Ideally, the leader prepares for the meeting and selects an optimal time for all parties. It is important for the leader to separate the problem from the people involved, stay focused on the issues, and work on one at a time. The next step is to identify available options and attempt to mediate a solution. The goal is to agree on an outcome based upon fair, objective criteria. Evaluating the outcomes by checking back in with the parties is important. Keep in mind cultural differences and individual conflict resolution styles:

- Avoidance
- Accommodation
- Coerciveness
- Competition
- Compromise
- Collaboration

MEMBER OF A PROFESSION

The nurse leader is accountable for the ongoing acquisition of knowledge and skills to effect change in healthcare practice and outcomes in the profession. The leader examines trends in health care, attends professional meetings, and participates by sharing knowledge and information. Nurse leaders participate in the process of translating relevant and current clinical research into patient care. Participating in panels and presenting posters, symposia, or clinical outcome data aids the process of translation.

Lifelong Learner

The nurse leader actively pursues new knowledge and skills as her or his role and needs of the healthcare system evolve. Research utilization is a practice standard and an essential component of evidence-based practice (see Chapter 11). Keeping up with every change in psychiatric–mental health nursing is impossible; however, attending professional conferences and workshops, reading selected journals, and maintaining specialty certification are a few ways of remaining competent in our highly complex healthcare environment.

REFERENCES

American Association of Colleges of Nursing. (2007). *White paper on the education and role of the clinical nurse leader.* Retrieved January 14, 2009, from www.aacn.nche.edu/publications/whitepapers/ClinicalNurseLeader07.pdf

American Hospital Association. (2008). *A patient care partnership. Understanding expectations, rights and responsibilities.* Retrieved January 14, 2009, from http://www.aha.org/aha/issues/Communicating-With-Patients/pt-care-partnership.html

American Nurses Association. (2001). *Code of ethics for nurses with interpretive statements.* Retrieved January 14, 2009, from http://nursingworld.org/MainMenuCategories/ThePracticeofProfessionalNursing/EthicsStandards/CodeofEthics.aspx

American Nurses Association and the National Council of State Boards of Nursing. (2007). *Joint statement on delegation.* Retrieved January 14, 2009, from https://www.ncsbn.org/1056.htm

Brenner, P. (1984). *From novice to expert: Excellence and power in clinical nursing practice.* Menlo Park, CA: Addison-Wesley.

Institute of Medicine's Committee on Crossing the Quality Chasm: Adaptation to Mental Health and Addictive Disorders. (2006). *Improving the quality of health care for mental and substance-use conditions: Quality chasm series.* Washington, DC: The National Academies Press.

Institute of Medicine's Committee on Quality of Health Care in America. (2001). *Crossing the quality chasm: A new health system for the 21st century.* Washington, DC: The National Academies Press.

Institute of Medicine's Committee on the Work Environment for Nurses and Patient Safety. (2004). *Keeping patients safe: Transforming the work environment for nurses and patient safety.* Washington, DC: The National Academies Press.

Marquis, B., & Huston, C. (1992). *Leadership roles and management functions in nursing.* Philadelphia: J. B. Lippincott.

National Council of State Boards of Nursing. (1997). *The five rights of delegation.* Retrieved January 14, 2009, from www.ncsbn.org/fiverights.pdf

Research

Karan Kverno, PhD, PMHNP-BC, PMHCNS-BC

RESEARCH: SCOPE OF PRACTICE

The *Psychiatric Mental-Health Nursing Scope and Standards of Practice* (2007) specifies the role of research in nursing practice. The registered nurse:

- Utilizes best available evidence, including research findings, to guide practice decisions.
- Actively participates in research activities at various levels appropriate to the nurse's level of education and position, including:
  - Identifying of clinical problems specific to nursing research
  - Participating in data collection
  - Participating in formal committees
  - Sharing research findings with peers and others
  - Conducting research
  - Critically analyzing and interpreting research for application to practice
  - Using research findings in the development of policies, procedures, and standards of practice
  - Incorporating research as a basis for learning

FIVE STEPS OF EVIDENCE-BASED PRACTICE

Evidence-based practice consists of finding and using the best available evidence to guide our practice. That doesn't mean that the nurse has to conduct research studies to find the evidence, but it does mean that nurses are charged with keeping up to date and *utilizing* the best available evidence to guide practice and *evaluating* patient care outcomes (see Box 11–1).

The five steps of evidence-based-practice are:
1. Ask an answerable clinical question.
2. Collect the most relevant and best evidence.
3. Critically appraise the evidence.
4. Synthesize and integrate with professional experience, patient preferences, and values in making a practice decision or change.
5. Evaluate the practice decision or change.

Box 11–1. Essentials of Evidence-Based Practice

Research: The systematic gathering of information to gain, expand, or validate knowledge about health and responses to health problems

Research Utilization: The use of research findings in practice

Outcome Evaluation: The final activity of evidence-based practice that examines whether the application of evidence-based care resulted in an improvement or met expected treatment goals

---

Step 1. Ask an Answerable and Relevant Clinical Question

Both research and research utilization require the identification of a relevant clinical question. The "PICO" (Oxman et al., 1993) mnemonic can be used to guide the process of developing a question that can be answered by reviewing the literature:
• Patient population
• Intervention or area of interest
• Comparison interventions
• Outcome measures

Step 2. Collect the Most Relevant and Best Evidence

It is not enough to simply read one glowing article about a particular intervention and take it as evidence. Reviewing the literature for the most relevant and best evidence is a systematic process that involves searching for:
• Systematic reviews of the literature or as many single studies as possible
• Best practice guidelines
• Clinical pathways

The *best evidence hierarchy* (see Box 11–2) can be used to evaluate the strength or validity of the identified literature.

Box 11–2. Best Evidence Hierarchy

1. Systematic review or meta-analysis of all randomized controlled trials (RCTs), or evidence-based clinical practice guidelines based on systematic reviews of RCTs
2. At least one experimental/RCT
3. Quasi-experimental studies (controlled trials without randomization)
4. Case-control and cohort studies
5. Systematic reviews of descriptive and qualitative studies
6. Single descriptive or qualitative studies
7. Opinions or reports of authorities or expert committees

Adapted from *Evidence-based practice in nursing and healthcare: A guide to best practice* by B. Melnyk, & E. Fineout-Overholt, 2004, Baltimore: Lippincott Williams & Wilkins.

Searching the Research Literature

Systematic reviews represent the evaluation and synthesis of ALL available literature on a particular topic, and are therefore considered to be the highest level of evidence. Systematic review articles can be found by searching online databases. The Cochrane Library, of the Cochrane Collaboration (available online at www.cochrane.org), provides a database of current systematic review articles on all of the major mental disorders. The Cochrane Collaboration is dedicated to the dissemination of up-to-date information to inform evidence-based practice.

Randomized controlled trials (RCTs), especially if they have been replicated, are considered to be strong evidence because of the way the studies are designed. RCTs control variables (such as age, race, gender, comorbidities, etc.) in determining participant eligibility. Participants are randomly assigned to the group getting the intervention of interest (e.g., the drug) or to the group getting either the usual treatment or placebo. Controlling variables and randomly assigning the participants, rather than letting them pick their own group, minimizes the possibility that the two groups are somehow different prior to the intervention and makes findings of posttreatment differences much more interpretable. RCTs can answer research questions about cause and effect.

Quasi-experimental studies compare two naturally occurring groups of interest. For example, a researcher could implement a new treatment (e.g., communal dining) on one unit of a treatment center, but not another, and then compare patient satisfaction between the two units. The problem with quasi-experimental designs is that the differences between groups could be the result of some unknown variable (e.g., staff turnover).

Case control studies are retrospective observational studies used to determine factors that may contribute to a medical condition by comparing patients who have the condition with individuals who do not. Case control studies have helped us understand certain risk factors (e.g., smoking) associated with the development of illnesses (e.g., lung cancer); however, they are subject to confounding because the researcher has little knowledge of other factors that may have influenced the outcome.

Cohort studies are prospective observational studies that are used to examine variables that might be relevant to the development of a condition. For example, a researcher might choose to study children of depressed mothers to determine whether they develop any behavioral or emotional problems over time. The problem with this type of design is again, the lack of control and the possible effects of some unknown variable. Studies examining relationships between variables cannot answer cause and effect questions.

Single descriptive (cross-sectional) or *qualitative* studies add to our knowledge about a condition, but must be replicated to provide reliable evidence. For example, if the prevalence of schizophrenia is found to be 1% in many different countries, and in urban and rural sites, this would provide strong evidence for a prevalence of 1%, but it would not provide us with any further information concerning the contributions of nature versus nurture, and so on. Qualitative studies are important in helping us understand the lived experience of illness. They are frequently based upon the analysis of interview data and the identification of themes.

Expert opinions are also important and need to be considered in relation to available evidence.

Searching for Best Practice Models

Evidence-based models of care are best practices. Best practice models require the synthesis and translation of relevant research findings into guidelines for practice.

Practice guidelines provide detailed specification of the methods and procedures for treating an identified healthcare problem. These represent the synthesis of systematic literature reviews and knowledge into a set of guidelines that can be used for prevention, case-finding, diagnosis, and treatment. Many different agencies publish best practice guidelines for treating individuals with psychiatric disorders, including the National Guideline Clearinghouse (www.guideline.gov), the American Psychiatric Association, and the Agency for Healthcare Policy and Research.

Clinical pathways are practice guidelines that identify key clinical processes and corresponding timelines. They are generally developed by healthcare professionals within inpatient settings and serve as a shortened version of the multidisciplinary care plan. Clinical pathways include the following specifications (Stuart, 2009):

- Identification of target population based on diagnoses (DSM-IV or nursing) conditions, treatments, interventions, or behaviors.
- Expected outcome described in a measurable, realistic, and patient-centered way.
- Specified treatment strategies and interventions.
- Documentation of patient care activities, variances, and goal achievement. This might be in the form of checklists.

Step 3. Critically Appraise the Evidence

Individual research study reports are usually organized in the following order. The title is very brief and refers to the population of interest and major variable(s). The abstract is a brief summary with approximately one sentence describing each section of the paper. The literature review provides the background for the study, the conceptual framework, and the hypotheses to be tested. The methods section describes the participants, the instruments, and the procedure. The intervention or manipulated variables are labeled "independent" and the outcome variables are called "dependent." The results section reports the findings. The discussion section presents the researchers' interpretations of the findings. The references section includes all cited studies.

We evaluate the *strength* of the evidence by the study design, using the best evidence hierarchy (Box 11–2). We evaluate the *quality* of the evidence from individual studies based upon sample size, experimental control, and the conclusions of the findings. If we are evaluating the evidence of a systematic review, we would additionally want to note whether the reviewed studies found consistent results. Table 11–1 provides a method for rating the strength and quality of research evidence.

Table 11–1. Strength and Quality of Research Evidence Rating Scheme

Level	Strength of Evidence/Design
I	Evidence obtained from an experimental study/randomized controlled trial or meta-analysis of RCTs
II	Evidence obtained from a quasi-experimental study
III	Evidence obtained from a nonexperimental study, qualitative study, or metasynthesis

Grade	Quality of Research Evidence
High	Sufficient sample, adequate control, and definitive conclusions. Consistent results and recommendations*
Good	Sufficient sample, some control, with fairly definitive conclusions. Reasonably consistent results and recommendations*
Low/Major Flaw(s)	Insufficient sample size, inadequate control, conclusions cannot be drawn. Little evidence with inconsistent results*

*The criterion of consistency is used when evaluating multiple studies (e.g., systematic review). Adapted from *Johns Hopkins nursing evidence-based practice model and guidelines* by R. Newhouse, S. Dearholt, S. Poe, L. Pugh, & K. White, 2007, Indianapolis: Sigma Theta Tau International.

Sample Size
The bigger the sample, the more generalizable the findings. A general rule is that a sample size of 30 or more is necessary for generalizable results, but the number of participants needed to interpret findings is actually based upon the number of variables in the study and the type of statistical analysis.

Control

The more control over the independent variable, the more interpretable the findings. Descriptive studies do not exercise any control. RCTs exercise the most control, with one group receiving the intervention and another serving as a placebo or comparison control group.

Conclusions

The conclusions that we draw from research are dependent upon the design of the study and the questions asked or hypotheses tested. In descriptive studies, we organize and summarize data. Descriptive studies tend to be hypothesis-generating. Studies using inferential statistics allow us to test hypotheses and make conclusions about a population from a sample. A result is considered to be significant if it is unlikely to have occurred by chance. Statistical significance does not necessarily mean that a result is clinically relevant.

Statistics

There are two major types of statistics: *descriptive* and *inferential*. The level of measurement determines or constrains the types of descriptive and inferential statistics that may be applied to the variable (see Table 11–2).

Table 11–2. Levels of Measurement

Level	Definition	Examples	Statistics
Nominal	Categorical, named variables	Group 1, Group 2, Group 3 Red, white, blue Race, religion	Count Frequencies
Ordinal	Rank order	Rankings 1st, 2nd, 3rd Grades A, B, C Likert and psychometric scales	Count Frequencies
Interval	Equal differences between values, but no true starting point	Days, education, temperature (a temperature of zero is not an absence of temperature)	Can be added, subtracted, multiplied and divided.
Ratio	Ratios between measurements are meaningful with a set zero point	Age, weight, number of children, etc.	Can be added, subtracted, multiplied and divided. Ratios are meaningful.

Descriptive statistics are used to describe the basic features of the data in a study. The majority of nursing studies are descriptive. When reporting descriptive findings, the researcher reports numerical values that summarize, organize, and describe the observations.

- *Frequency:* How often a particular finding occurs. Frequencies are useful for describing nominal or ordinal data.
- *Mean:* A measure of central tendency derived by summing all scores and dividing by the number of participants. Means can be found for interval and ratio data.
- *Standard deviation:* A measure of the distance of a measure from the group mean. Based upon the formula for calculating the standard deviation, approximately 68% of the scores will fall within one standard deviation from the mean, approximately 95% will fall within two standard deviations, and approximately 99% will fall within three standard deviations (see Figure 11–1). Interval and ratio level data are normally distributed.
- *Variance:* A measure of variation derived by squaring each standard deviation in a set of scores and then taking the mean of the squares. The larger the variance, the greater the dispersion of scores.

Figure 11–1. The Normal Distribution

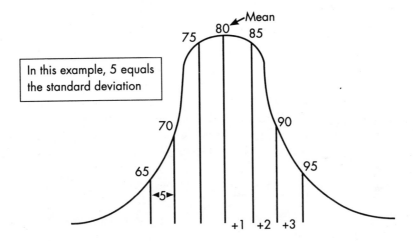

Inferential statistics are used to reach conclusions that extend beyond the immediate data alone. They are used to infer something about a population based upon sample data. For example, a researcher might want to make a judgment of the probability that a new medication will be efficacious for treating individuals with bipolar depression. The use of an experimentally controlled research design, interval or ratio level variables, and the calculation of inferential statistics would allow the test of a null hypothesis of no difference between the two populations of interest.

- *Probability:* A qualitative statement of the likelihood that an event will occur. A probability of 0 means that the event is certain not to occur; a probability of 1 means that the event will occur with certainty.
- *Probability value (P-value):* With inferential statistics, we test the hypothesis that there will be no difference between groups (e.g., the experimental and control group). A P-value for a hypothesis test is the probability of obtaining, by chance alone, a value of the test statistic as extreme or more extreme than the one actually computed when the null hypothesis is true. The convention for judging the *statistical significance* of a P-value is the significance level that we set. In most studies, a P-value less than 0.05 is considered statistically significant.

- *Analysis of variance:* A set of statistical procedures designed to compare two or more groups of observations. It determines whether the differences between groups are due to experimental influence or chance alone. A simple t-test can be used to test differences between two groups.

Are the Conclusions Valid?

In other words, are the conclusions right or true? Types of validity include the following:
- *Internal validity:* Is there a relationship between the intervention and the outcome? Did the treatment cause the outcome?
- *External validity:* Can we *generalize* the findings? Was the sample large enough, representative enough, and so on?

Are the Conclusions Reliable?

In other words, were the measures consistent?
- *Test/retest:* Assuming there is no change in the underlying condition (e.g., trait or personality), does the measurement tool obtain the same result on repeated measures?

Step 4. Synthesize and Integrate With Professional Experience, Patient Preferences, and Values in Making a Practice Decision or Change

Nurses have a great deal of practice-based knowledge based upon experience. Professional experience and knowledge should be considered in combination with the utilization of research-based knowledge to determine the best plan of care for individual patients. In line with the Institute of Medicine's call to transform the mental health care system, treatment plans should be patient-centered, that is, respectful of and responsive to individual patient preferences, needs, and values, and ensuring that patient values guide all clinical decisions (IOM, 2004).

Research findings cannot be helpful unless they are translated into practice. The length of time between the completion of research studies and the translation of their findings into clinical practice is often many years. The Agency for Healthcare Research and Quality and other national agencies are working to accelerate the impact of health services research on direct patient care, but we can all help by keeping abreast of new developments in the field of psychiatric care.

Step 5. Evaluate the Practice Decision or Change

The last step of evidence-based care is to evaluate the response to the practice decision or change in care. Change can only be measured if baseline levels are known. For example, to evaluate the efficacy of a preventive exercise plan on depression, it would be essential to take baseline as well as periodic depression surveys. To measure response to care, outcomes indicators must be specified.

Characteristics of Good Outcome Measures:
- Measurable, reliable, valid (see Box 11–3 for examples of standardized psychiatric measurement tools in the public domain)
- Suitable to the population of interest

- Not overly costly to collect
- Sensitive to changes within or across individuals
- Nondirectional: People may not change in the direction expected

Types of Outcome Indicators:
- *Clinical outcomes:* Health status, relapse, recurrence, readmission, number of episodes, symptomatology, coping responses, high-risk behaviors, incidence reports
- *Functional outcomes:* Functional status (e.g., DSM-IV Global Assessment of Functioning), social interaction, activities of daily living, occupational abilities, quality of life, family relationships, housing arrangements
- *Satisfaction outcomes:* Satisfaction with treatment, treatment outcomes, treatment team or organization
- *Financial outcomes:* Cost, revenue, length of stay, use of resources

The use of standardized psychometric outcome measurement tools is essential for identifying the quantity and quality of change. Box 11–3 lists examples of some of the psychometric outcome measurement tools that are available in the public domain. Standardized outcome measures allow us to make evidence-based care a continuous part of everyday practice.

The development of a national database of psychiatric core standardized screening and evaluation measures will be useful for quality improvement, benchmarking, accountability, decision-making, accreditation, and research. The Joint Commission, together with the National Association of Psychiatric Health Systems (NAPHS), the National Association of State Mental Health Program Directors (NASMHPD), and the NASMHPD Research Institute, Inc. (NRI), developed a set of core performance measures for hospital-based inpatient psychiatric services (HBIPS) that are available for use.

Box 11-3. Examples of Standardized Measurement Scales for Psychiatric Practice

General Symptom Measures
- Brief Psychiatric Rating Scale (BPRS; Overall, 1988)

Alcohol Withdrawal
- Clinical Institute Withdrawal Assessment for Alcohol Withdrawal or (CIWA-A; Shaw et al., 1981)

Cognitive Functioning
- Mini Mental State Examination (MMSE; Folstein et al., 1975)

Depression
- Hamilton Rating Scale for Depression (HAM-D; Hamilton, 1960)
- Cornell Scale for Depression in Dementia (CSDD; Alexopoulos et al., 1988)

Abnormal Movement/Extrapyramidal Symptoms
- Abnormal Involuntary Movement Scale (AIMS; Guy, 1976)

All listed tools are in the public domain and can be used in clinical practice. These are only examples. There are many other measurement scales available.

ETHICAL CONSIDERATIONS IN RESEARCH

Ethics involves doing what is right. All investigators or individuals involved in research studies must take and pass a required test on the protection of human subjects based on the the *Belmont Report* (National Commission for the Protection of Human Subjects of Biomedical and Behavioral Research, 1979). This requires researchers to meet the criteria of:

- *Beneficence* (do no harm)
- *Respect for human dignity* (right for self-determination)
- *Justice* (fair treatment and nondiscriminatory selection)

Evaluation of Research Ethics

- Were women, children, minorities, elderly included? In the past, most healthcare research was conducted with White males. Determine whether best evidence for excluded subgroups is available.
- Were there conflicts of interest on the part of the investigators? Drug companies fund the majority of RCTs. Was there inappropriate involvement of research sponsors in the design and management of the RCT? Drug company sponsors stand to profit from favorable outcomes.
- Was there a publication bias in the dissemination of results? Were financial incentives given? Are the bar or line graphs depicting the results based upon using equivalent dosages of comparison drugs, with equivalent age groups, and so on?

Institutional Review Boards

Institutional review boards (IRBs) exist within most healthcare and academic institutions to review all studies to ensure that:

- Risks to subjects are minimized.
- Subject selection is equitable and without coercion.
- Informed consent is obtained and documented (see below).
- Data and safety monitoring plan is implemented when indicated.

Informed Consent

According to the U.S. Office for Human Research Protections (OHRP; www.hhs.gov/ohrp), the Code of Federal Regulations (CFR) requires that certain information be provided to research participants before they participate in a study, including:

- A description of the purpose and procedures
- A description of any reasonably foreseeable risks or discomforts
- A description of any benefits (usually none)
- A disclosure of appropriate alternative procedures or courses of treatment
- A statement describing the extent, if any, to which confidentiality of records and identity will be maintained
- A description of any treatments or compensations for injury
- An explanation of whom to contact with questions
- A statement that participation is voluntary and that refusal to participate, or decision to discontinue participation, will involve no penalty or loss of benefits to which the participant is otherwise entitled

REFERENCES

Alexopoulos, G., Abrams, R., Young, R., & Shamoian, C. (1988). Cornell scale for depression in dementia. *Biological Psychiatry, 23,* 271–284.

American Nurses Association. (2007). *Psychiatric–mental health nursing: Scope and standards of practice.* Silver Spring, MD: Author.

Committee on Quality of Health Care in America, Institute of Medicine. (2001). *Crossing the quality chasm: A new health system for the 21st century.* Washington, DC: National Academies Press.

Folstein, M., Folstein, S., & McHugh, P. (1975). "Mini-mental state." A practical method for grading the cognitive state of patients for the clinician. *Journal of Psychiatric Research, 12,* 189–198.

Guy, W. (1976). *ECDEU: Assessment manual for psychopharmacology* (DHEW Publ. No. 76-338). Washington, DC: Department of Health, Education, and Welfare, Psychopharmacology Research Branch.

Hamilton, M. (1960). A rating scale for depression. *Journal of Neurology, Neurosurgery and Psychiatry, 23,* 56–62.

Institute of Medicine. (2004). *Health literacy: Aprescription to end confusion.* Washington, DC: Author

The Joint Commission. (2008). *Specifications manual for national hospital inpatient quality measures: Hospital-based inpatient psychiatric services core measurement set. Verson 2.0.* Oakbrook Terrace, IL: The Joint Commission.

Melnyk, B., & Fineout-Overholt, E. (2004). *Evidence-based practice in nursing and healthcare: A guide to best practice.* Baltimore: Lippincott Williams & Wilkins.

National Commission for the Protection of Human Subjects of Biomedical and Behavioral Research. (1979). *The Belmont report.* Retrieved January 14, 2009, from http://www.hhs.gov/ohrp/ humansubjects/guidance/belmont.htm

Newhouse, R., Dearholt, S., Poe, S., Pugh, L., & White, K. (2007). *Johns Hopkins nursing evidence-based practice model and guidelines.* Indianapolis: Sigma Theta Tau International.

Overall, J. (1988). The Brief Psychiatric Rating Scale (BPRS): Recent developments in ascertainment and scaling. *Psychopharmacology Bulletin, 24,* 97–99.

Oxman, A., Sackett, D., Guyatt, G., & Evidence-Based Medicine Work Group. (1993). Users' guides to evidence-based medicine. *Journal of the American Medical Association, 270,* 2093–2095.

Shaw J., Kolesar G., Sellers E., Kaplan H., & Sandor, P. (1981). Development of optimal treatment tactics for alcohol withdrawal, I: Assessment and effectiveness of supportive care. *Journal of Clinical Psychopharmacology, 8,* 382–389.

Stuart, G. (2009). *Principles and practice of psychiatric nursing* (9th ed.). St. Louis, MO: Mosby Elsevier.

Appendix A. Review Questions

1. Which of the following statements is true about differentiated practice roles?
   a. Levels are determined by each State Board of Nursing.
   b. Levels are determined by education and expected skills.
   c. Levels are determined by a particular nurse's job position.
   d. Levels are administratively determined by the nurse's practice setting.

2. Monica, a nurse on the mental health unit, is working with a drug-addicted client who is manipulative and denies she has a drug problem. Monica finds herself becoming very annoyed with this client's behavior and wanting to distance herself from her. This is a clinical example of
   a. Transference
   b. Countertransference
   c. Mirroring
   d. Introjections

3. Betty is 16 years old and is expecting her first child within a few weeks. She is unmarried, hopes to finish her high school education, and later marry her boyfriend. Betty is very excited and feels confident that she can be a good mother. In working with this client from a developmental perspective, which of Erikson's stages of psychosocial development should be MOST appropriate as a consideration?
   a. Identity vs. role confusion
   b. Intimacy vs. isolation
   c. Generativity vs. stagnation
   d. Purpose vs. function

4. Sam is a 9-year-old who is the last one picked to play on school sports teams, has trouble handing in his assignments, and difficulty making friends. According to Erikson's theory, Sam's difficulty in mastering this stage of development can lead to
   a. A poor sense of self-identity
   b. Feelings of inferiority
   c. Mistrust of self and others
   d. A sense of guilt and stagnation

5. An adolescent is admitted to the hospital with a history of drinking beer daily, lying, stealing, and not being able to control his behavior. Using Freud's approach to personality development, this adolescent's behavior reflects a defect related to
   a. Animus
   b. Ego
   c. Id
   d. Superego

6. The mother of an acutely ill schizophrenic patient says, "I can't understand why this is happening to me. Why me, why does he act this way?" Which of the following active listening responses would be most appropriate to use with her to help her talk about her anguish at her son's illness?
   a. Paraphrasing
   b. Reflecting
   c. Summarizing
   d. Silence

7. The main goal of therapeutic communication is to
   a. Encourage assertive behaviors and learning
   b. Facilitate socialization and prevent patients from feeling lonely
   c. Help patients to clarify issues and develop different perspectives
   d. Provide new information about ways to cope with mental symptoms

8. Jane is upset about her father not coming to visit her in the hospital. "He just doesn't care about me, or he would be here." An appropriate response by the nurse might be:
   a. "That's a very common feeling."
   b. "He'll be here later, wait and see."
   c. "It sounds like his not coming today is painful."
   d. "Why don't you give him a call and find out where he is."

9. Mary has been counseling a disturbed teenager for several weeks. There have been several breakthroughs in the sessions, which is gratifying for both nurse and patient. The teenager asks Mary for a hug, because she feels close to her. What would be the most appropriate response from Mary?
   a. Giving the teenager a hug
   b. Asking the teenager why she wants a hug
   c. Explaining to the teenager that she too appreciates the closeness, but can't give her a hug
   d. Explaining about boundaries, and how boundaries make the relationship safe

10. If a patient has a current Global Assessment of Functioning of 55, with the highest GAF during the past year of 80, this tells us that the patient is
    a. Currently functioning with little psychological impairment
    b. Demonstrating more psychological symptoms currently than in the past year
    c. Demonstrating fewer psychological symptoms currently than during the past year
    d. At some danger of hurting self or others

11. An evidence-based screening tool for detecting potential alcohol abuse is the:
    a. CAGE
    b. BDI
    c. MMPI
    d. AIMS

12. What is primary difference between Axis I and Axis II disorders?
    a. Axis II disorders tend to be chronic and less responsive.
    b. Axis II disorders tend to present with more florid symptoms.
    c. Axis II disorders are usually the focus of clinical attention.
    d. Axis II disorders are an indication of environmental stress.

13. JD lost his job 4 months ago and has had difficulty finding a new job. He continues to look for work, but reports symptoms of anxiety, depression, and insomnia. He does not meet criteria for major depression or any of the specific anxiety disorders. He is requesting stress management. The best nursing diagnosis for him is:
    a. Social isolation
    b. Anxiety
    c. Ineffective coping
    d. Bereavement

14. A 17-year-old girl is referred to the school nurse due to poor school performance, including restlessness, agitation, and difficulty coping with minor stressors. The prior school year she served as class president and her school performance was excellent. What would be the best next step in evaluating the problem?
    a. Make a nursing diagnosis of ineffective coping.
    b. Recommend peer group counseling.
    c. Refer her to the school counselor.
    d. Screen for depression and SI/HI.

15. The nurse assigned to monitor a violent patient in the seclusion room fails to take his vital signs at the prescribed intervals because the patient seemed to be sleeping and the nurse didn't want to disturb him. The patient suffered a stroke in the seclusion room. A key standard by which this nurse's actions would be judged as negligent in a court of law would involve
    a. The actions that a reasonable and prudent nurse with similar education and experience would take in a similar situation
    b. The nature of the physician's orders and agency policy
    c. The other responsibilities the nurse had at the time, and whether this offered a sufficient rationale
    d. Whether the patient's stroke could have been avoided, if the vital signs had been taken.

16. An ethical dilemma exists when
    a. There are two choices, both of which are potentially justifiable.
    b. There is no consensus about the appropriate course of action.
    c. An action is required, but the parties disagree on when it should be implemented.
    d. One choice is appropriate, but it is more difficult or costly to implement.

17. When is the most appropriate time to begin the process of discharge planning for a patient admitted to an inpatient psychiatric facility?
    a. Once the discharge order is written
    b. Once the insurance company is alerted and has approved the discharge
    c. Within 24 hours of the planned discharge
    d. Upon the patient's admission to the inpatient unit

18. Jay, a chronic schizophrenic, took a piece of watermelon rind and stuffed it in his mouth. Within less than a minute, he was turning blue and choking, and subsequently choked to death before he could be revived. This death warrants being recorded as
    a. An incident report
    b. A sentinel event
    c. A risk management variance
    d. Quality improvement divergence from norms

19. Which action by the nurse could potentially compromise a patient's confidentiality when the nurse uses computerized patient records?
    a. Giving a password to a trusted colleague who has forgotten hers
    b. Logging off all computer screens as the nurse is about to leave the computer
    c. Changing passwords at regular intervals
    d. Preventing other coworkers from viewing the computer screen

20. The _____ engages (sets off) the body's fight-or-flight response.
    a. Thalamus
    b. Optic nerve
    c. Hypothalamus
    d. Cerebral cortex

21. Movement disorders such as bradykinesia and hyperkinesia suggest
    a. Disease or impairment of the basal ganglia
    b. The early stages of Alzheimer's disease
    c. A dietary deficiency
    d. A tumor or stroke affecting the cerebellum

22. Early trauma or abuse may produce vulnerability to depression in adulthood via a dysregulation of
    a. Endogenous opioids
    b. The hypothalamus-pituitary-adrenal (HPA) axis
    c. Acetylcholine
    d. The alarm response

23. Which of the following problems is most closely associated with dysfunction of the frontal lobes?
    a. Loss of vision
    b. Loss of the sensation of touch
    c. Loss of balance
    d. Loss of executive functions

24. The most common cause of residual effects of benzodiazepine sedative hypnotics is
    a. Depressed respirations
    b. Half-life of the drug
    c. History of drug abuse
    d. Tolerance to the drug

25. A 22-year-old college student presented to the ER with hypertension (BP = 200/110), tachycardia, cramping, hyperreflexia, and myoclonus. He was taking phenelzine and had been out to a restaurant with friends. What is the most likely food/drink that could have interacted with the medication?
    a. Cucumbers
    b. Grapefruit juice
    c. Red wine
    d. Peanuts

26. "Dry as a bone, red as a beat, hot as a hare, blind as a bat, and mad as a hatter" describes the symptoms of
    a. Anticholinergic toxicity
    b. Serotonin syndrome
    c. Neuroleptic malignant syndrome
    d. Lithium toxicity

27. With conventional antipsychotics, the higher the potency,
    a. The lower the risk for EPS
    b. The higher the risk for EPS
    c. The lower the risk of dystonia
    d. The higher the risk of sedation

28. A 43-year-old man with schizophrenia who has been taking clozapine presents with a fever and sore throat. The nurse would be prudent to consider
    a. Tardive dyskinesia
    b. Serotonin syndrome
    c. Agranulocytosis
    d. Akathisia

29. A group member comments, "I never knew so many people thought like I did." This is an example of which one of Yalom's curative factors?
    a. Imitative behavior
    b. Universality
    c. Corrective reenactment of the primary family group
    d. Instillation of hope

30. On the first day of mixed-gender group therapy, a woman reveals intimate personal details of her developmental history. The other group members make no comments in support of her. The best explanation for the group's behavior is that
    a. The leader has not indicated that this is appropriate behavior.
    b. Members need to develop trust before responding.
    c. The other members do not like her.
    d. Members can't relate because their developmental history is different.

31. Which of the following reinforcement schedules is the most effective in maintaining behavior change from a behavioral therapy perspective?
    a. Continuous
    b. Fixed interval
    c. Variable interval
    d. Variable ratio

32. A family seeks counseling for their son. During an interview session, the mother, sitting next to her son, answered all three questions you addressed to her son. The behavior observed is an example of
    a. Poor communication
    b. Enmeshment
    c. Disengagement
    d. A family rule

33. Julie is a victim of domestic abuse, but doesn't feel she can leave her husband because of the children and her financial dependence on him. She tells the nurse, "This time it will be different; Jack has promised that he will not hurt me again if I come home, and I really believe him." The nurse's most appropriate response would be
    a. "In most cases of abuse, the abuser is likely to continue with episodes of violence and promises of transformation."
    b. "You are the best judge of his sincerity, so you probably can count on his love for you."
    c. "I wonder if it would be helpful for you to look at the ways in which you might have provoked his wrath."
    d. "As your husband grows older, the abuse is likely to lessen anyway because of his maturity."

34. The level of prevention associated with screening for depression is
    a. Primary
    b. Secondary
    c. Tertiary
    d. Targeted

35. Which of the following individuals would have the highest risk for suicide?
    a. A chronic schizophrenic patient
    b. A young adult who has just lost a significant relationship
    c. A psychotic patient with command hallucinations
    d. A patient with borderline personality disorder

36. John is a new patient on the unit with serious anger management issues. The nurse is helping him to develop strategies to prevent his inappropriate anger outbursts. The learning objective "The patient will develop a realistic plan for appropriately handling his anger impulses" falls under which one of Bloom's taxonomy classifications?
    a. Analysis
    b. Evaluation
    c. Knowledge
    d. Synthesis

37. Discussing the pros and cons of change and providing information about solutions is associated with which one of Prochaska's stages of change?
    a. Precontemplation
    b. Contemplation
    c. Preparation
    d. Maintenance

38. Which of the following is an example of a "teach-back" teaching format?
    a. "Can you tell me how you would know that your medication is working for you?"
    b. "I'd like to give you some brochures to help you in case you forget anything."
    c. "Please feel free to call me if you have any questions after the session."
    d. "Would you be willing to talk about your experience with medication with some of the other patients on the unit?"

39. An expert nurse clinician exercises what kind of power?
    a. Coercive
    b. Legitimate
    c. Referent
    d. Expert

40. Legitimate power is
    a. Power given by others
    b. Power granted by title
    c. Power gained by information
    d. Power gained by expertise

41. On a busy work day, the RN delegates the task of assisting a newly arrived patient to the community room for lunch. Why is this wrong?
    a. The task is not within the nursing scope of practice.
    b. There has been no assessment of patient needs.
    c. The delegating nurse is not competent to make delegating decisions.
    d. The nursing assistive personnel do not have the appropriate knowledge.

42. What nursing task cannot be delegated to an unlicensed nursing assistant?
    a. Taking vital signs, height, and weight
    b. Assistance with personal hygiene
    c. Socialization activities
    d. Evaluation of response to care

43. The individuals selected for measurement in a study are called
    a. Sample
    b. Small group
    c. Variable
    d. Population

44. The level of measurement identified by a depression severity scale ranging 1–30 is
    a. Nominal
    b. Ordinal
    c. Interval
    d. Ratio

45. In a published research study, where in the manuscript would you find a step-by-step description of how the study was carried out?
    a. Abstract
    b. Literature review
    c. Methods
    d. Discussion

Appendix B. Answers to the Review Questions

1. **Correct Answer: B.** Differentiated nursing practice roles are structured on the basis of education, experience, and competence.

2. **Correct Answer: B.** Countertransference refers to the therapist's unconscious feelings and reactions to a client based on personal projections.

3. **Correct Answer: A.** According to Erikson, the primary developmental task of adolescence is identity vs. role confusion.

4. **Correct Answer: B.** Industry vs. inferiority is the psychosocial crisis associated with the childhood years, 6 to 12 years. Children in this stage are concerned with themselves as individuals, and in being good at what they are doing.

5. **Correct Answer: C.** According to Freud, the id functions in the irrational and emotional part of the mind as the pleasure principle.

6. **Correct Answer: B.** Reflection focuses on the emotional aspects of a communication and best allows the client to identify feelings he or she may have in relation to a situation.

7. **Correct Answer: C.** The primary goal of therapeutic communication is to help individuals and families clarify issues and develop different, more productive perspectives on ways to manage their lives.

8. **Correct Answer: C.** Using a reflective listening response helps the client clarify important feelings in relation to a particular situation.

9. **Correct Answer: D.** Clients need to know that the relationship they have with the nurse is non-exploitive. Therapeutic boundaries help ensure the safety of the relationship for both client and nurse.

10. **Correct Answer: B.** The Global Assessment of Functioning is scored from 1 (persistent danger of severely hurting self or others) to 100 (superior functioning). A change from 80 to 55 indicates that the patient has gone from having transient symptoms in the past year to having moderate psychological symptoms.

11. **Correct Answer: A.** The CAGE is a screening tool for alcohol-related problems. A "yes" response to any one of the 4 questions indicates the need for further assessment. A "yes" response to 2 questions indicates probable alcohol abuse or dependence.

12. **Correct Answer: A.** Though Axis I disorders are usually the focus of clinical attention, Axis II disorders are more chronic and are thought to be less responsive to treatment. These include the personality disorders and mental retardation.

13. **Correct Answer: C.** Nursing diagnoses identify problems that can be treated by nursing interventions. Although JD does have some anxiety symptoms and may be grieving the loss of a job, the primary focus of nursing care will be to help JD cope more effectively with stressful life transitions.

14. **Correct Answer: D.** An accurate diagnosis depends upon a complete evaluation. The next step in diagnosing the patient is to screen for depression and other life events (e.g., abuse) that may be responsible for her change in coping.

15. **Correct Answer: A.** Judgments about nursing negligence usually are made on the basis of what actions a reasonable and prudent nurse with similar education and experience would do in a similar situation.

16. **Correct Answer: A.** An ethical dilemma occurs when there is an apparent conflict between two or more potentially justifiable courses of action in which one would preclude acting on the other.

17. **Correct Answer: D.** Discharge planning should begin when the patient is first admitted to the inpatient unit.

18. **Correct Answer: B.** The Joint Commission requires that any unexpected occurrence involving death or serious injury be reported as a sentinel event.

19. **Correct Answer: A.** Under HIPAA regulations, healthcare providers are charged with protecting all personal identifiable information about their patients. Passwords for any private information about a patient should not be shared with anyone else.

20. **Correct Answer: C.** Under conditions of stress, the hypothalamus triggers the activation of the autonomic nervous system (ANS). The fight-or-flight response refers to the acute stress response resulting from activation of the sympathetic branch of the ANS.

21. **Correct Answer: A.** The basal ganglia are important brain structures for initiating voluntary movement. Involuntary movements (dyskinesias) and slow movements (bradykinesia) reflect a problem in the basal ganglia or their dopaminergic pathways.

22. **Correct Answer: B.** There are two major stress pathways in the brain. One is the fight-or-flight response of increase peripheral epinephrine (adrenaline). The other is a slower and less perceivable response that results from stimulation of the hypothalamus-pituitary-adrenal (HPA) axis. In prolonged situations of chronic stress, the acute

stress response may subside, but the chronic stress pathway may continue to secrete excess cortisol. When trauma occurs in childhood, the hypothalamus may become dysregulated and secrete excessive cortisol in response to stressors. Chronically elevevated levels of cortisol are a possible mechanism for the development of depression.

23. **Correct Answer: D.** Executive functions, such as decision making, planning, and organizing, are dependent on the prefrontal cortex, the most anterior portions of the frontal lobes.

24. **Correct Answer: B.** Benzodiazepine drugs given at night for insomnia may impair next-day performance if the half-life of the drug is long, and/or if the dosage is too high. Some benzodiazepines, such as flurazepam, have active metabolites that substantially increase the half-life of the drug and can result in daytime sleepiness, psychomotor impairment, and memory problems.

25. **Correct Answer: C.** Monoamine inhibitors (MAOIs) inhibit the enzyme (MAO) that breaks down monoamine neurotransmitters (i.e., dopamine, norephinephrine, serotonin) once they have been pumped back into the presynaptic cell. While taking MAOIs, certain foods and alcohol that are high in the amino acid tyramine (aged, pickled, processed) can cause a severe hypertensive crisis and should be avoided.

26. **Correct Answer: A.** Anticholinergic toxicity is a potentially fatal condition characterized by skin that is hot, dry, and flushed, blurred vision, and CNS effects (hallucinations and delirium). Death can result from respiratory depression caused by the blockage of muscarinic cholinergic receptors. Many of the psychiatric drugs have anticholinergic side effects, especially the tricyclic antidepressants and phenothiazine antipsychotics. These should be used cautiously in older adults and in patients taking multiple drugs with anticholinergic properties.

27. **Correct Answer: B.** Conventional antipsychotics with high potency have a stronger D2 receptor blockade than those with low potency, thereby decreasing dopamine levels in the nigrostriatal pathway. This can result in drug-induced extrapyramidal side-effects involving movement, including parkinsonism (tremor, bradykinesia, rigidity), dyskinesias, and akathesia.

28. **Correct Answer: C.** Agranulocytosis, a potentially life-threatening side effect of Clozapine, is defined by a low total white blood count (WBC), and is characterized by sore throat, fever, malaise, or bleeding. Because of the higher risk of agranulocytosis with clozapine treatment, WBCs are measured weekly for the first 6 months, then less frequently. If WBC drops below 2000 cells/mm^3, the drug is discontinued.

29. **Correct Answer: B.** Yalom refers to the discovery that other people have the same problems and thoughts that a particular group member does as universality.

30. **Correct Answer: B.** Since the group is in the formative stage of group development, sharing of deep feelings is not appropriate. Group members need to know and trust each other before feeling comfortable sharing intimate details of their life.

31. **Correct Answer: D.** Variable ratio in which a reinforcer given after correct responses is given on an uneven rather than set number of correct responses works best for maintaining behavior.

32. **Correct Answer: B.** Enmeshment (structural therapy concept) occurs when family members are so close emotionally that they answer for one another and are too heavily involved in a family member's life.

33. **Correct Answer: A.** The pattern of domestic abuse is one in which tension escalates, followed by an abusive event and then a "honeymoon phase" in which the abuser is very solicitous and repentant. The cycle of abuse is repetitive and predictable.

34. **Correct Answer: B.** Screening activities for people with high risk or in the early stage of disease are associated with secondary prevention.

35. **Correct Answer: C.** Suicide is a complication of schizophrenia, bipolar disorder, major depression with psychotic features, and schizoaffective disorder. Particularly at risk are individuals with command hallucinations.

36. **Correct Answer: D.** Bloom's taxonomy uses the term *synthesis* to describe pulling together a plan to accomplish identified goals.

37. **Correct Answer: B.** Contemplation is the stage in which people are deciding to make changes, possibly within the next 6 months. Discussing pros and cons of making changes and providing information about solutions can help clients decide in favor of making a change.

38. **Correct Answer: A.** Teach-back methodologies ask patients to repeat back training information for the purpose of assessing understanding and identifying gaps in understanding. Gaps in information can be re-taught.

39. **Correct Answer: D.** Expert power is leadership gained through knowledge, expertise, or experience.

40. **Correct Answer: B.** Legitimate power is derived from a person's organizational title or position rather than from a personal quality.

41. **Correct Answer: B.** Although the nurse can delegate the task to a nursing assistant, a thorough assessment must be completed before sending a newly admitted patient into the community area with other patients.

42. **Correct Answer: D.** The nurse may delegate nursing tasks, but not nursing practice. The nurse takes the responsibility and accountability for evaluating the patient's response to care.

43. **Correct Answer: A.** The sample consists of the individuals selected to participate in a research study. Randomized selection and assignment to groups helps assure that the sample represents the actual population from which they came.

44. **Correct Answer: B.** Psychometric scales are usually measured at the ordinal level. A score of 30 on the Beck Depression Inventory (BDI) is definitely higher than 15 but is not necessarily exactly half as high in terms of meaningful symptoms.

45. **Correct Answer: C.** The methods section identifies the steps that were taken to carry out the study, including the tools and time frames for measuring outcomes. An interested researcher should be able to replicate the methods based upon the written description.

Index

Note: Page numbers in *italics* indicate tables, figures, and boxes.

About the Authors

Elizabeth Arnold, PhD, RN, CS-P, is a retired associate professor in psychiatric mental health nursing and the former graduate behavioral specialty coordinator for the University of Maryland School of Nursing. She maintains a private practice as a psychiatric clinical specialist. Prior to her work at the university, Dr. Arnold served as the in-service coordinator for Noyes Division at St. Elizabeths Hospital in Washington, DC. She is a graduate of Georgetown University and received her master's degree from Catholic University in psychiatric mental health nursing. Her PhD is in Human Development from the University of Maryland. Dr. Arnold is an ELNEC-certified trainer in end-of-life care, and was the primary investigator on three funded training grants from HRSA related to the development of graduate studies in behavioral health nursing. She also was the recipient of two Helene Fuld training grants. Currently, she serves as the non-physician representative on the Montgomery County Advisory Committee on Mental Health, and as the mental health liaison to the Alcohol and Drug Abuse Advisory Committee for Montgomery County.

Dr. Arnold has presented her research on mid-life women entering the second half of life and caring from the graduate student perspective at national and international conferences. A related poster received an APNA award for excellence in Nursing Research in 2004. She is co-author of *Interpersonal Relationships: Professional Communication Skills for Nurses,* currently in its 5th edition. This text was selected as an AJN Book of the Year in 2000 and 2007, as well as being listed in Brandon Hill as a recommended text for nursing libraries. She has written book chapters and articles related to burnout, stress, dementia, caring, and other psychiatric nursing topics. Recently she presented a 2-day seminar on the DSM-IV-TR to the psychiatric nursing fellows at the NIH Clinical Center.

Karan S. Kverno, PhD, PMHNP-BC, PMHCNS-BC, Assistant Professor at University of Maryland School of Nursing, has been teaching psychiatric and mental health nursing to undergraduate and graduate students since 1998. She is certified by ANCC as a Psychiatric Mental Health Clinical Specialist and Nurse Practitioner, and has practiced in psychiatric mental health nursing since 1985. Dr. Kverno was awarded the first Blaustein post-doctoral Fellowship in Psychiatric and Mental Health Nursing at Johns Hopkins University School of Nursing. Her research and recent publications focus on improving non-pharmacological treatments for the distressing psychiatric and behavioral symptoms associated with dementia.